Masters of Disasters

An irreverent look at the other side of America's lifesavers.

A compilation of the stories, truths, poems and just fun stuff that helps us keep our sanity in the often chaotic, pressure filled world of Emergency Services.

Compiled over the years and edited by:
Chris St,John and Lou Jordan
with illustrations by:
Bruce Bollinger

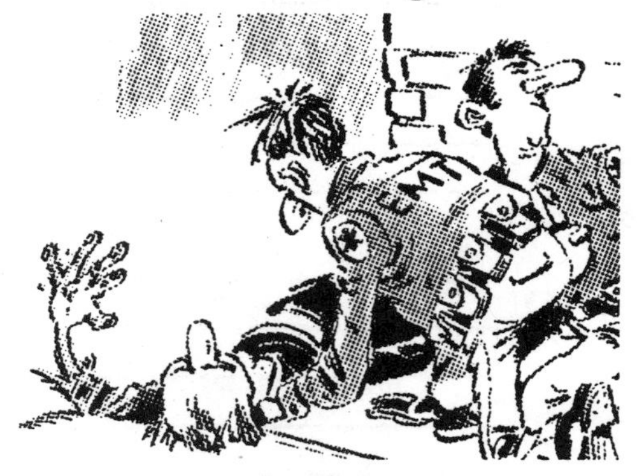

Published by:
Emergency Training Associates
PO Box 164
Union Bridge, MD. 21791

Distributed by:
www.EMSBooks.com
Your on line Emergency Services Bookstore

Celebrating 20+ years of serving Emergency Services personnel with low prices,and fast service.

Contact us at
1-800-367-0382
or
Fax 410-775-0691

Recognizing the special needs of you, our readers, and in appreciation of you purchasing this book we are pleased to provide you with this unique added feature at no additional cost.

Personal Information Page

This page is for you to collect and save important information, promising phone numbers and autographs.

Fast Food Joints ______________________________

____

____

____

____

____

____

____

____

____

Promising Phone Numbers

____

____

____

____

____

____

____

____

Autographs ______________________________

____

____

____

____

____

____

Other ______________________________

Personal page of:____

Placing your name here might make your partner feel a bit guilty when they steal this book. (sign in ink)

Premise:

Nearly all of this content has been collected from various sources over the years. The sharing of our own brand of humor continues to offer us a way of achieving mental relief from the seriousness of our tasks. With the recent surge in internet communications a number of these tales have resurfaced via the Internet and other anonymous sources of contributions.

Some of these tales, or urban legend's as they are now called, are classics that seem to continuously tuned up or modernized and resurface time and time again. Some are new and will undoubtably become tomorrow's classics.

As you read through this book you may be reminded of similar tales from the past....this may be an indicator that you like those tales are aging gracefully.

You may have heard some of them recently and be surprised to find that they are just stories that have come to life once again with a hint of local flavor added.

Take the time to relax and laugh at yourself as well as your counterparts as you go through this book, and rest assured that we have compiled this information to laugh with each other...not at each other.

The participants in compiling the material in this book have made an effort to give credit to the appropriate individuals when they have been identifiable. Any previous copyright infringement is not intentional,

The text is written in the gender specific form in which the contributions were collected. The authors, and certainly the individuals involved with this compilation, recognize the contribution of both sexes and the roles that they play in Emergency Services. Likewise, some ethnic references may appear...these are reproduced as received, and may be changed to reflect most any of our diverse ethnic population..

Please feel free to mentally change the gender or ethnic references as you enjoy this book, I am sure you will find that the material could easily apply to many.

Dedication

This book is dedicated to our families and families of the thousands today, who wear a badge or perhaps have a title that goes with their chosen role as a "helper of people in need".

The families that stand behind and support these individuals often sacrifice a normal life to allow their loved ones to do what they do. Supporting those who take on the task of "lifesaver" often means missed appointments, late meals and many unscheduled changes in their lives as well. These sacrifices often go unrecognized. In many instances the "lifesavers" could not be there without this understanding and support.

It is also dedicated to the un heralded thousands of potential lifesavers stand ready to respond when they get the call, give everything they have, even on occasion, as much as their life. This is most often done for someone they have never met before nor may never see again.

They are the thousands whose eyes have witnessed the very worst in this world, but have never surrender their beliefs, hope or honor. They continue to come back for more, making the difference in many lives and making this world a better place, one call at a time.

These are perhaps the people we owe the most to, but it is far to infrequent when we hear a greatful "thank you" to a police officer, a firefighter, a medic, nurse or doctor. Yet, as you read this, they are there taking time away from their own families, And because of their special dedication they will be there when you or someone sends out a call for help.

America is blessed to have "lifesavers" that follow tradition, belief and caring. These people continue to give so much of themselves to make this world safer for us, our children, and the millions across this great nation.

So sleep well America, you couldn't be in better hands.

Chris & Lou

Printed in USA,
2000
ISBN# 1-887321-01-2

Preface

From the earliest days of firefighting and responding to medical or other emergencies, field responders have developed a sense of irreverent humor, largely as a defense mechanism to cushion their fear, anxieties, and compassion for life.These people prepare for the next possible disaster that could occur. It could be a disaster for one person or many. They may crawl into a twisted steel cage that once was a fine automobile to search for signs of life among its occupants, look for people in a burning home or respond to a scene where violence has been reported.

With an overwhelming desire to sustain the flame of life from the last flicker of a spark that is near spent, they cope on a daily basis with variables that few people can tolerate. Without humor, many of us would not be able to keep our sanity and still deal with death, serious illness, and the tragedies of others. It has often been said we quite often "deal with people at their worst".

Most people can avoid and deny awareness of the human response to injury or illness. It's too overwhelming for most people to think about. We in Emergency services can't aviod it, because, our job is partly to treat this human response. We face it, head on, and we see it far too often.

Much is written in the psychiatric literature addresses the emotional damage caused by unshared secrets. These secrets are often about abuse, alcoholism or a family member's inappropriate behavior. However, it is not just the information that does the damage. It is the isolation that comes from keeping the secret. The walls of defense. The fear of exposure.

Humor relieves stress. It does this by sharing our secrets in a safe environment. Acknowledging our responses to what we see and know, Often laughing about our feelings, we frequently find out other health care providers feel that way too, It makes our feelings OK. It makes us OK. It helps us face our jobs. It helps us stay in the profession.

While I do relish those slang terms that aptly characterize patients or situations not otherwise easily described, I am wary of pejorative or denigrating terms. I am especially interested in providing terms that clarify a clinical presentation, or in national or regional differences in nomenclature. These are not intended to be offensive. All in all we speak and understand the same language....

While there is no intent to hurt or belittle anyone, the terms and language used in the presentations found in this book may not be condoned by those without an understanding of our special, way of sharing our laughter. They just wouldn't understand, but if you are one of us...... you will.

Chris St.John
Silver Spring, Maryland
May, 2000

Lou Jordan
Union Bridge, Maryland
May, 2000

Christopher St.John, MSEd, NREMTP has been involved with EMS systems since 1974. He serves with a Baltimore-Washington DC fire department and enjoys mentoring young probies. Over the decades he has been accumulating the wisdom of the ER, courage of the streets and gems from our brothers and sisters. No claim to unique authorship exists except where noted.

Lou Jordan became an Army Medic in 1960 and has accumulated thousands of hours listening to and telling stories like those in this book. Having worked at the Local, State and National level of Emergency Services he often believes he has heard or seen it all...then life proves him wrong...he laughs a lot. as he observes the funny side of Emergency Services. He says "it is most fitting that we have chosen the humorous artist of Cracked and Mad Magazine fame to poke fun at ourselves"

Cartoonist Bruce Bolinger began his freelance studio in the secluded mountains of western Pennsylvania in 1976. Since then he has produced artwork and cartoons for over 500 books and 50 greeting cards. 25 year highlights include his wife and partner, Valerie, two offspring, and a quarter-acre of pet cemetery. Bruce was the assistant to the late, great Don Martin of Mad and Cracked magazine fame. He is still turning ink to gold and is currently a monthly regular with Cracked magazine.

To send contributions for inclusion in future editions please mail them to:

Masters of Disasters
Emergency Training Associates
PO Box 164
Union Bridge, MD. 21791
or e-mail to:
MD@EMSBooks.com

Enclose your name and address. If your material is the first received and used we will send you a free copy of the next edition.

If there were a neat way to categorize this material we would call this page the.....

Table of Contents

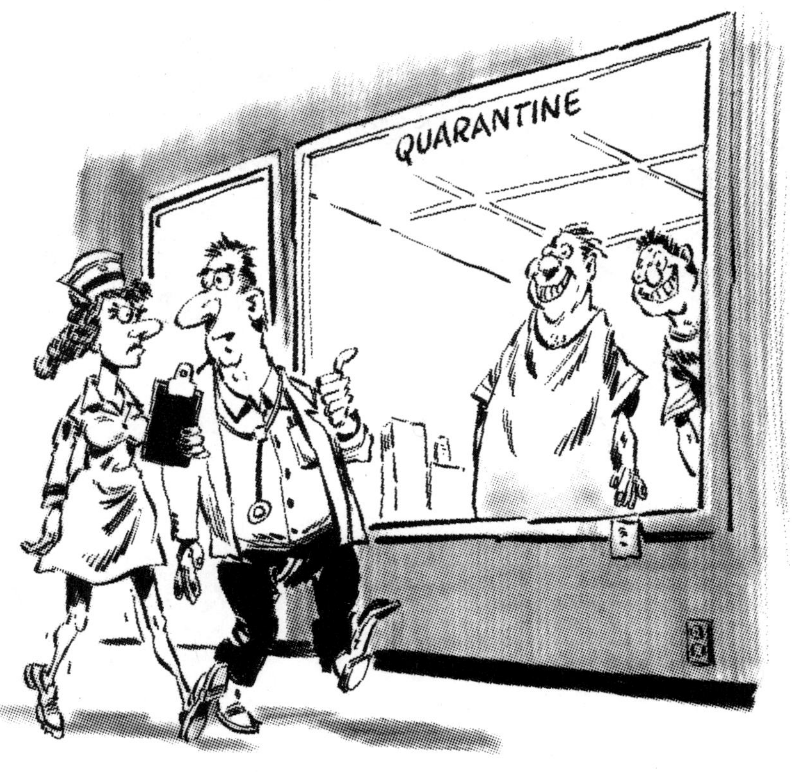

..and to the left is the infectious grin ward..

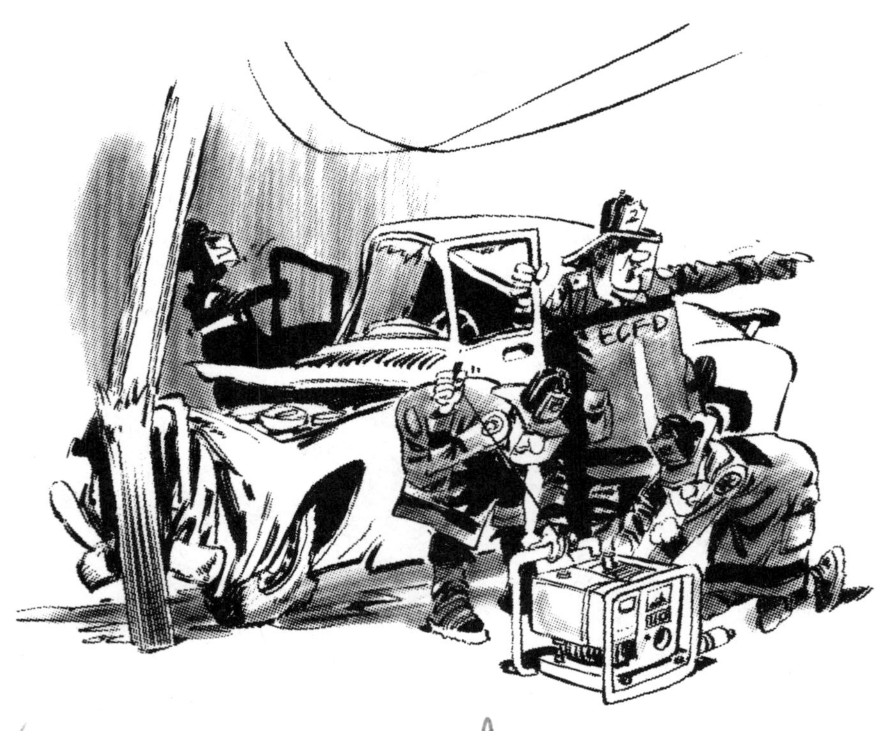

“ Bring the small saw, I want to seperate her from her attorney.”

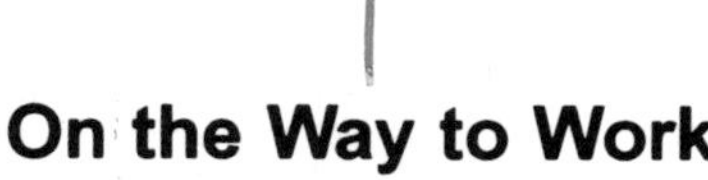

On the Way to Work

License Plates Seen on the Street

CD8D	An Anesthesiologist
ISD8EM	Another gas passer
O2BCD8D	And another
SQLAPS	Aesculapius "God of Healing"
	Geez, is he vain or what??
ATHDOC	An Athletic Trainer
CPR MD	A Cardiologist
ECGDXRX	A Cardiologist
NTG PRN	A Cardiologist
A4RENXT	"A Ferrari next" - a Cardiac Surgeon
1TOETAG	A County Coroner
2TH MD	A Dentist
B4DKCME	A Dentist
TOOF DR	A Dentist
SAY AAH	A Dentist
FT DKY	A Children's Dentist
CME4DK	Another Dentist
2 3PAIR	An Oral Surgeon
OPN WYD	Another Oral Surgeon
ITCH DR	A Dermatologist
911EMER	A Fire Dispatcher
911 WIFE	The Dispatcher's wife
STAT2ER	An ER physician
TRMADOC	An ER physician
STATMD1	An ER physician

ERDOC2B	An ER Resident
MRGENCY	Plate on ER nurse's car
RD DR	A Fire Surgeon's other car
IRESQ	A Firefighter
MZ CHF	The Fire Chief's Wife
2Z RESQ	A Truckee at the Station
1FYTFYR	A Volunteer Firefighter
FIREHWK	A Firefighter
BODYFXR	My Internist
IXMN8U	Another Internist
CULATR	A Mortician
MBALMED	An Embalmer
ITSTYME	A 1968 Cadillac Hearse
RM41MR	Another Hearse
THE END	A Mortician's blue Cadillac
APGAR 10	An OB/GYN
STORK1	An Obstetrician
TZVECL	An Opthamologist (the 20/20 line on the eye chart)
DR IIII	An Optician (Dr Four Eyes?)
DR IBALZ	An Optometrist
STR8NR	An Orthodontist
ETOH PRN	Seen in a hospital parking lot
NTG EMT	A Paramedic
NAHRTBT	A Paramedic
NTG PRN	Another paramedic
CARPE PM	An EMTs car (Seize the night??)
BONEFXR	An Orthopedic Surgeon
BONE MD	Another Ortho Doc

BXDXRX	“Biopsy, diagnose, prescribe” - Obviously a Pathologist
PILPUSR	On a Pharmacist’s 1990 Corvette
TMRZAPR	“Tumor zapper” - A Radiation Oncologist
DNTSMKE	A Respiratory Therapist
DOC4JOX	A Sports Medicine specialist
STAT2OR	A Surgeon
GUT-SEE	A Surgeon
BIG BUX	A Surgeon’s Ferrari 308
BOXDOC	(Self explanatory)
UNOPCME	“U no P, C me” - a Urologist
PP DR	A Urologist
UP4ME	Another Urologist
PETDOC	A Veterinarian
HRTZAPR	Plate on Chris’s Jeep 4x4

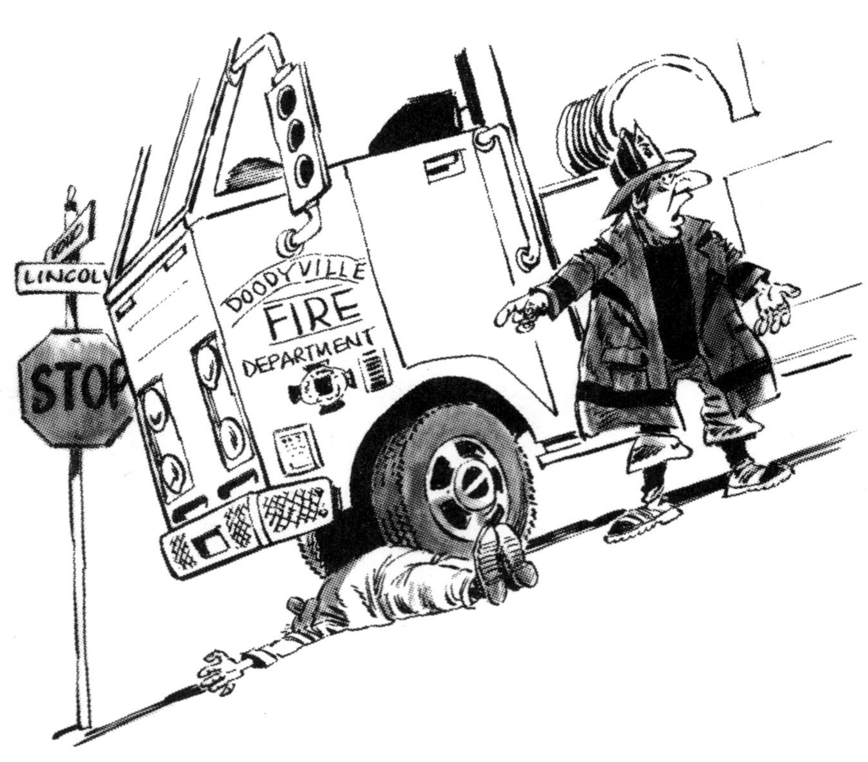

"Charlie, bring one more Probie for the other wheel."

Morning Line-Up

Chief Page's Testament of 1918

**WHEN A PERSON JOINS
A FIRE DEPARTMENT**

THE ACT OF BRAVERY HAS ALREADY BEEN ACCOMPLISHED.

**WHAT YOU DO AFTER
THAT IS ALL IN
THE LINE OF DUTY.**

What is a Fireman?

He's the guy next door - a man's man with the memory of a little boy.

He has never gotten over the excitement of engines and sirens and danger.

He's a guy like you and me with warts and worries and unfulfilled dreams. Yet he stands taller than most of us.

He's a fireman.

He puts it all on the line when the bell rings.

A fireman is at once the most fortunate and the least fortunate of men.

He's a man who saves lives because he has seen too much death.

He's a gentle man because he has seen the awesome power of violence out of control.

He's responsive to a child's laughter because his arms have held too many small bodies that will never laugh again.

He's a man who appreciates the simple pleasures of life - hot coffee held in numb, unbending fingers - a warm bed for bone and muscle compelled beyond feeling - the camaraderie of brave men - the divine peace and selfless service of a job well done in the name of all men.

He doesn't wear buttons or wave flags or shout obscenities.

When he marches, it is to honor a fallen comrade.

He doesn't preach the brotherhood of man.

He lives it.

Author Unknown

Who is EMS?

Somewhere in the realm of society, located just between the security of sanity and the neurosis that precedes psychosis, we find a group of individuals who seek out those that cling to life and death by a slender thread. These people are those who make up what is known as EMS.

You may find these people located in various positions within the county, prepared for the next possible disaster that could occur, hindered in their travel only by the natural obstacle of daily traffic.
No other group of humanity can carry so many items in pockets that are strategically located in optimal positions on the body. Perhaps you will find scissors, bandages, tape, chapstick, combs or essential life sustaining items, but one thing that is certain, the last paycheck, if they are paid for their work, has long since met it's demise and will not be found here.

With an overwhelming desire to sustain the flame of life from the last flicker of a spark that is near spent, these people cope on a daily basis with variables that few people can tolerate. When things go right, the public loves them, the newspapers and TV ignore them, and life goes on.

These individuals come from all walks of life with few standing on common ground until they meet in the surroundings of the insanity of the streets. Then they all seem to pull together with each needing the others to lean on for support. They occasionally share the stories that can create a flurry of mixed emotions.

What kind of people are these?

They are the people to whom you may need to trust with the life of yourself or loved ones.
They walk tall, but may crawl into the twisted steel wreckage that moments ago was an automobile as they search for signs of life among its occupants.
They are the calm voice on the other end of the telephone when it seems as though your world is crashing around you.

These people are often the last to win the respect of their public and the first to be sought after by lawyers who critically challange actions made on the spur of the moment, in an environment of absolute chaos.

THESE ARE THE MEN AND WOMEN OF EMS......

An EMT Prayer

God ... grant me the ability to give emergency care
With skillful hands, knowledgeable mind
and tender love and care.
Help me deal with everything,
when lives are on the line
to see the worst, administer aid, and
ease a worried mind
So help me as I go today,
accept what fate may be
Touch these hands, use this mind,
Help this EMT.
Amen.

Battling The Beast

Wearing blue uniforms, we sit
sometimes for days, laughing,
eating, joking...waiting
for one sound, a siren
that transforms us.

We abandon our armchairs for overcoats
of canvas and for rubber boots,
their armor heavy and hot.

Instead of trading jokes we relay
directions, and orders, and shout
reports of the status of the enemy—
"FLAMES ARE VISIBLE"

Fear and excitement grip the hearts
of the freshest rookie to the oldest veteran
as we jump into the steel Trojan horses
perfect from polishing,
washing, checking over and over —
we pray that we have made no mistakes.

The driver navigates
the craft through the city streets
he knows as well as his family,
dodging when possible those
that get in the way, hoping those
he can't avoid will see him first,
the spot the enemy from blocks away—
the phoenix rises far above the trees,
licking the sky.

We arrive at the scene, and again
the battle cry is heard—
"FLAMES ARE VISIBLE"

Smoke fills the air and our lungs
as we approach, hoses snaking,
crisscrossing, coming to life
as they surge with water
from yellow and red hydrants
that suddenly become grotesque
heads of Medusa.

We kick open the doors, rubber
from our boots leaving a print
melted by the heat, and trickling
over bubbling paint.

Orange liquid flames roll
through the building, slithering
up and over the walls, breathing
in and out with each puff of air.

With swords of water we charge
and the war begins.
We battle—9 or 10 against one —
seemingly great odds.

But, as soldiers, we will win,
emerging from the battlefield victorious
as we always do, and eventually,
we'll retire to our armchairs,
thanking God that this time nobody
was hit by the enemy Fire...

EMS Levels of Care

(or "What the initial after the "EMT" stands for)

With the beginning of EMS in the early 60"s the term used was EMT-A which designated Emergency Medical Tecnician-Ambulance. Since that time and with the proliferation of governmental bureacuracy and medical oversite we have experienced a nationwide proliferation of various and often redundant "brands" of EMS level's of care. With each change comes an oportunity for new and exciting patches and titles.Using up all the letters in the alphabet was so quickly accomplished, that now it is not uncommon to find that combinations of numbers and letters are used to designate the specialty areas of EMS.

To help clarify some of these alphabet EMT's we asked for our resident researcher to clarify the following: alphabet designations.

by Lisa Larson, NREMT-P, Gaithersburg-Washington Grove VFD

EMT-A: Ambulance—The person who most resembles an ambulance. Either they look like one, or they sound like one.

EMT-B: Basic—They cannot do anything but the most minor skills. They are not supposed to think, just do.

EMT-C: Complicated—They can do everything, have done everything, and can handle even the most difficult situation.

EMT-D: Deaf—This person can only hear the tones/pager/partner when he/she wants to. This does not include during any meal or when their "favorite show" is on TV.

EMT-E: Egocentric—They are the only reason why the ambulance can get out the door. Without them, the ambulance service would fall apart.

EMT-F: Forgetful—They have to keep running back and forth to the ambulance for supplies/radio/whatever because they can't remember to bring everything at once.

EMT-G: "Gung-ho"—Runs to the ambulance with every call, is out the door carrying everything in sight before you put the unit in park, and has the patient treated before you can get your gloves on.

EMT-H: Hurler—Everytime they see blood, vomit, or feces, they hurl.

EMT-I: Idiot—This person never attends drills, never puts on gloves or other PPE, forgets about scene safety, and wouldn't know HazMat from butter.

EMT-J: Joker—Never lets 10 seconds go by without some smart-ass comment about something, be it your hair, the patient, the dinner, or whatever.

EMT-K: Killer—Can't touch a patient without the patient going downhill quickly. Also known as "Kevorkian."

EMT-L: Laid back—Walks everywhere, even in danger, doesn't let anything bother him/her, accepts whatever management puts onto them, including "mandatory overtime," This one makes Valium addicts look wired.

EMT-M: Mean—Never has anything good to say, plays cruel practical jokes, and causes more fights with patients and family than anyone you know.

EMT-N: Numbnuts—The guy (for obvious reasons male) who is in the bucket seat of the car with a gear shift in the middle and doesn't realize it until too late.

EMT-O: "Oh my God"—No matter what happens, good or bad, always tries to see the worst thing that could happen. A cut finger is always considered a "partial amuptation," or musculoskeletal chest pain is diagnosed as"the big one."

EMT-P: Paragod (or Paragoddess)—Walks on water, gives orders to God, is the only person in existence who knows (or could know) as much as they do.

EMT-Q: Quiet—The one who sits in the back of the unit, never saying a word, while the IV runs dry or the patient codes. They are always "afraid to bother you."

EMT-R: Return—Leaves the company for a "better position," then comes back, then leaves for "more pay," then comes back. You want to get rid of them permanently, but they keep coming back.

EMT-S: Shocker—The one who forgets to say "Clear" before defibrillating the patient.

EMT-T: Tipsy—Can't remember when his shift starts and happy hour ends.

EMT-U: Unconscious—The person who you try and try to wake up for the 0300 "sick person," but just can't arouse. So you drag them to the ambulance, and they wake up when you turn on the siren.

EMT-V: Vain—Can't pass a mirror without checking to see if they look as good in their uniform as they think they do. Always has a lint brush with them.

EMT-W: Whacker—Has a "police package" car, with 25 or more antennas, wears "EMT" t-shirts, pants, socks, and underwear, is never seen without a radio or two and at least 3 pagers, and will respond to every call in his/her personal vehicle "Code 3."

EMT-X: X-ray—Can "tell" that the cold is really pneumonia, can "tell" that the sprain is a break, and can see right through any skin/clothing/house/car to tell "exactly" what is wrong with the patient. Then "tells" the ER staff what he found (usually wrong).

EMT-Y:Yahoo—Wears the hat on backwards for everything, has his gun rack in the ambulance, and hasn't showered in a week, unless it has recently rained.

EMT-Z: Zebra—Wears white socks with his dark pants and white shirt.

You Know You met a Yahoo if ...

(Note: A "yes" answer to two or morel of the following statements makes it highly likely that the person you are talking to is a genuine "Yahoo" The higher the number of yes answers, the bigger the "Yahoo")

GENERAL YAHOO QUALIFICATIONS

He or she: His or her:

.. has multiple pagers for multiple stations

.. POV is a tactical command vehicle

.. talks more on the radio than a DJ does

.. knows every other station's alert tones by heart

.. entire wardrobe is station wear or off-duty stuff from the Galls catalog

.. sleeps with a scanner on all night, every night

.. overdue vehicle inspection sticker is covered by a Maltese Cross

.. washes the rigs every weekend, but has not washed his POV in years

.. parks in their home driveway backwards

.. thinks they are a "shoe in" for Chief/Captain

.. never misses watching "Rescue 911"

.. has multiple radio antennas on the POV

.. corrects Communications on how to dispatch units

.. has reflective striping on the POV

.. responds to a scene after recall

.. drives the apparatus like Mario Andretti

.. leaves her pager on open channel, all day

.. carries a pocket scanner

.. runs calls as a "service to the community"

.. subscribes to ALL fire and EMS magazines

.. responds to the station during alert tone tests

.. knows the names of every employee at the 7-11

.. doesn't drink alcohol because they "might get dispatched"

.. thinks they are "in the know", because they has a friend in gov ernment

.. has at least five different police hats, sweatshirts or t-shirts

FIREFIGHTER YAHOO QUALIFICATIONS

.. wears their badge everywhere

.. has 500 road flares in the trunk of the POV

.. fire decals obscure their rear vehicle window

.. argues with the Chief about apparatus placement

.. is studying to be a Paramedic, third attempt

.. has personalized road cones

.. thinks Sergeant/Lieutenant equals the rank of Chief

.. knows every police officer's name and thinks they are pals

.. wears a huge fire truck belt buckle

.. chases other companies trucks

.. knows everything about fire fighting, but can't pull hose

.. has watched Backdraft at least 50 times

.. has a Dalmation (or two)

.. owns an antique fire truck

.. names his dog "Sparky"

.. thinks water on magnesium "looks neat"

.. thinks dirt/holes in turnout gear is "Macho"

.. claims to have had sex on the hosebed "just like in Backdraft"

.. is an expert on which fire academy is best in the state

.. will not leave the structure when ALL-OUT is given

.. thinks high pressure is "just the thing" for interior attack

.. likes ony Neoprene

.. He thinks only "men" can fight fires

EMT YAHOO QUALIFICATIONS

..carries a stethoscope on the POV rear view mirror

.. KEDs the walking wounded

.. argues with ER doctors

.. pretends to be Johnnie Gage from "Emergency's Squad 51"

.. owns a velvet painting of John Gauge and Roy Desoto

..has a personal jump kit bigger than the one on the ambulance

..uses a 5-cell Mag light to check pupil response

..still carries a jawbreaker

.. owns a seatbelt knife

.. has a bumper sticker that says "I stop for all auto accidents."

.. personal vehicle has ever been mistaken for an EMS chase car.

..neighbors called the cops because they the scanner on in the car and they're tired of hearing every call being dispatched.

.. has underwear with little "stars of life" on it.

..thought a blood pressure cuff would be an excellent gift for Christmas.

..name is painted under the driver's side window on the amb ulance.

PARAMEDIC YAHOO QUALIFICATIONS
(To be used in addition to EMT Qualifications)

..considers it a big production when they starts an IV

..consider t's a bigger production when they intubate a patient

.. uses a cellular phone instead of the radio

.. wants to medevac everything

.. mutters to themself "great veins" when looking at complete strangers

..refers to a working code as a "GOOD CALL."

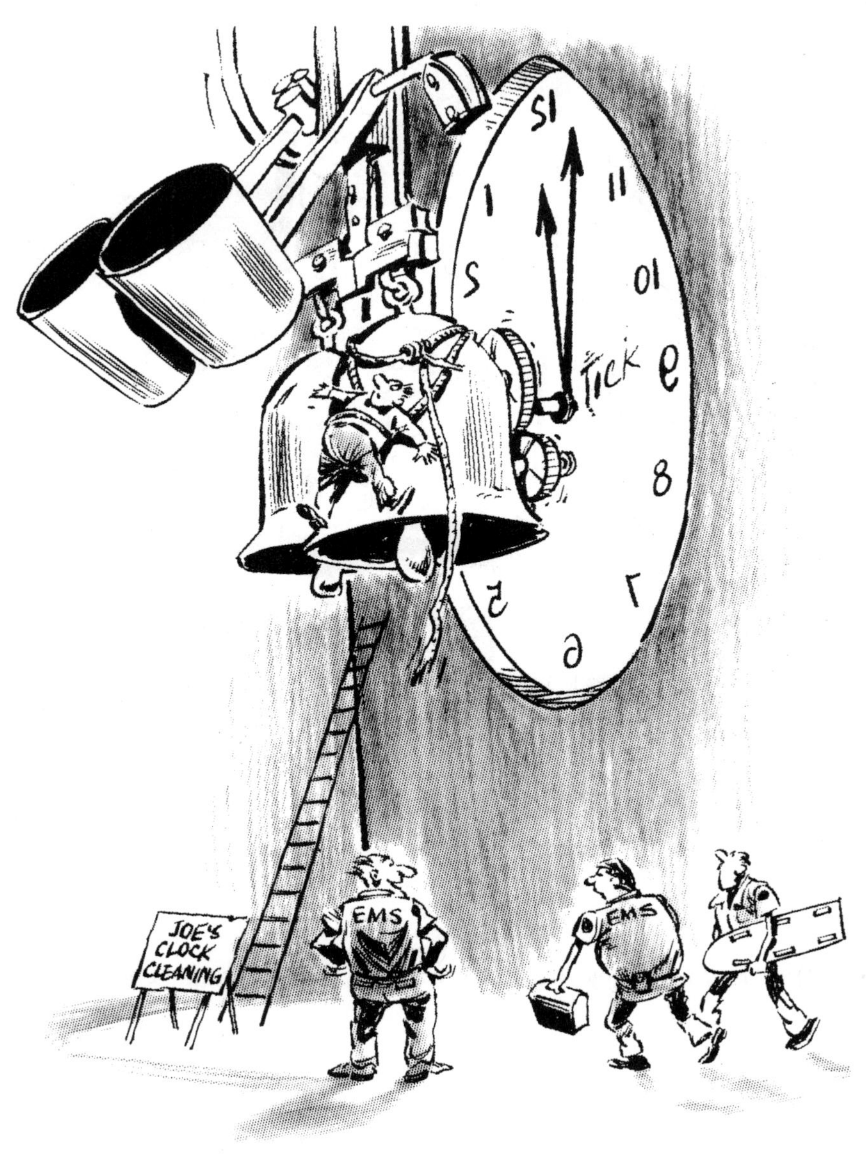

"Can you take this one? Looks like my shift will be done in a minute."

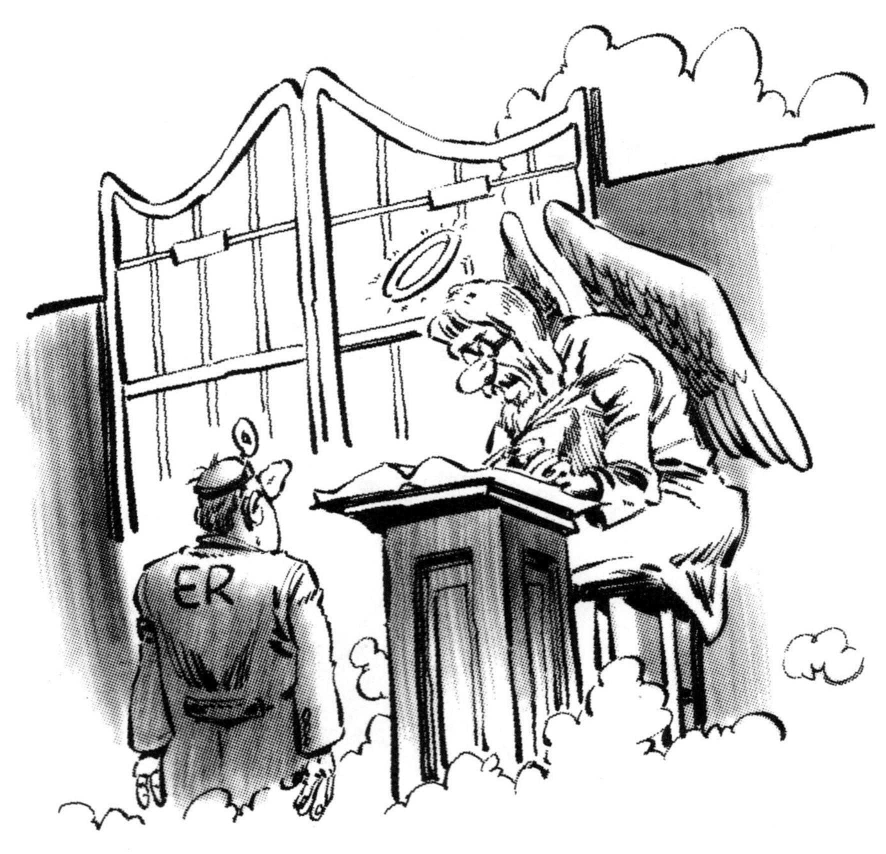

"Before you go anywhere I have to see your insurance card"

Continuing Ed

To My EMTs

Written by an unknown EMT Instructor

We've studied and practiced and studied some more,
and your friends say, "Gosh, you've become such a bore
with your talk of KEDs and something called MAST.
Will it ever be over? - How long will it last?"

"Quite a long time," you might have just said
for all of this knowledge is now in your head.
Not just to be there tucked deeply away,
but instead, for a purpose, to be used night or day."

Now you know there are 27 bones in the hand.
And you don't think of sea life when you hear SHRIMP CAN.
Burns you know, first - second - and third degree -
and you know that the patella is really the knee.

Ecchymosis is just a big word for bruise
and to get a pedal pulse you must first remove the shoes.
Diabetic coma is not at all like Insulin Shock.
Anterior hip dislocation - one foot in the boat and one on the dock.

Cover both eyes - the left and the right.
Don't forget to report all animal bites.
Don't induce vomiting if the culprit is lye,
and don't ever be ashamed to cry.

You can save someone's life with your knowledge and skill,
give someone hope - give someone the will
to keep on through even the darkest time
when life seems to have lost its rhythm and rhyme,
with the warmth of your smile and the touch of your hand,
with your eyes that say, "I understand."

More than medical skills I've tried to impart;
Remember, the brain cannot work without the heart.

Student Performance Objectives
Emergency Services Practical Examination

The following is a portion of a typical final exam, given to you in order to assist you in preparing for this year's exam. Instructions: Read each question carefully. Don t forget: neatness counts.

EMT SECTION

FIRST AID EXPLORER: You will be given a casualty presenting with an amputation of the left leg. Control hemorrhage and treat for complications. You have a trauma dressing and a blanket.

FIRST RESPONDER: You will be given a casualty presenting with an amputation of the left leg. Control hemorrhage and treat for complications. You have a sock.

EMT-B: You will be given a casualty presenting with an amputation of the left leg. Control hemorrhage and treat for complications. You have a band-aid.

CRT: You will be given a left leg presenting with an amputated casualty. Control hemorrhage and treat for complications. You have a Barry Manilow album.

EMT-P: You will be given a left leg presenting with an amputated casualty. Control hemorrhage and treat for complications. After 5 minutes the casualty will go into v-fib. The leg is pregnant. You have a toothpick.

FIREFIGHTING SECTION

FIREFIGHTING: You will be doused with gasoline and set on fire. You have a glass of water. Extinguish yourself within three minutes.

ADVANCED FIREFIGHTING: You will be doused in gasoline and set on fire. You have an empty glass. Extinguish yourself in two minutes.

HAZMAT: You will be doused in radioactive waste, then doused with petrol, then set on fire. Extinguish yourself, evacuate a suburb and identify which eastern european country the waste came from. You have four minutes. Points will be deducted if any local fauna develops a third set of legs.

RESCUE SECTION

EMT RESCUE: You will be given a casualty presenting with an amputated left leg. The casualty is hanging upside down from a car teetering on the edge of a cliff. The leg is floating down the river at the bottom of the cliff. Be back in 7 minutes with both parts.

POLICE RESCUE: As above, but the car must be issued with at least 7 traffic/defect violations.

FIRE RESCUE: As above, but everything is on fire.

MARITIME RESCUE: You receive a distress call from a ship identifying itself as the "Titanic". It seems to have encountered an iceberg. You have a canoe.

SUPPORT SERVICES SECTION

CRISIS COUNSELING: Your volunteer fire unit responds to a false alarm at what turns out to be Mr. T's residence. Explain to him that you have scratched his car with the fire truck. It is a Sunday morning at 3:23 am.

PUBLIC INFORMATION OFFICER SKILLS: Hold a press conference. Explain to the press that in three minutes, California will fall into the ocean. Stress that people should not panic. Points will be deducted if you forget any of the reporters' names during the question session.

VICTIM WELFARE: In ten minutes, 4000 homeless earthquake victims will be let into the room. Feed, clothe and house them. You have two McDonald's vouchers.

COMMUNICATIONS: A major incident has occurred in your local area. Organize inter-agency communications, an operations base, a dispatch system, and a satellite link to your national disaster agency. After five minutes, you will lose all power. You have a pigeon and a blunt crayon.

A Student's Last Rhyme Before the Registry Exam

In my car I sadly sit,
a damned crest-fallen chappy!
and own to you I feel a bit,
a little bit unhappy.

It really ain't the place nor time
to reel-off rhyming diction,
but yet I'll write a final rhyme
while waiting crucifixion.

No matter what the Registry decides,
pass, or fail.
I'll do my best when crucified
to finish off in style.

But I bequeath a parting tip
of sound advice for new recruits,
who come to do the final exam
to join an EMS group.

If you attempt the medic course
you really must study for it,
and if you don't want to get the boot
for pity's sake don't fail it.

So let's toss a cold one down our throats
before we do the test,
and toast the sweet instructor
we leave to teach the rest.

Wise Sayings and Rules to Live by

MURPHY'S LAW OF EMS

1) Anything that can go wrong will...
2) Murphy was an EMT.

STAIR'S MAJOR AXIOMS

The dead never get better, on the other hand they never get worse. Remember, asystole is a very stable rhythm.

THE BASIC LAW OF EMS

All emergency calls will wait until you begin to eat, regardless of the time.

COROLLARY 1.

Fewer accidents would occur if EMS personnel would never eat.

COROLLARY 2.

Always order food "to go".

THE BASIC BLS QUESTION

Can you walk? Have you tried?

FIVE GENERAL RULES

1) Pain never killed anyone
2) All bleeding eventually stops
3) All fevers eventually fall to room temperature
4) All patients eventually die
5) If you drop the baby, pick it up.

THE FIRST PRINCIPLE OF TRIAGE

In any accident, the degree of injury suffered by a patient is inversely proportional to the amount and volume of agonized screaming produced by that patient.

THE FIRST LAW OF AMBULANCE DRIVING

No matter how fast you drive the ambulance when responding to a call, it will never be fast enough, unless you pass a Police Cruiser, at which point it will be entirely too fast.

THE AXIOM OF LATE-NIGHT RUNS

If you respond to any MVA after midnight and do not find a drunk on the scene, keep looking — somebody is still missing.

THE LAW OF OPTIONS

Any patient, when given the option of either going to jail or going to the hospital by a police officer, will always be inside the ambulance before you are.

Cororollary 1. Any patient who chooses to go to jail instead of the hospital probably knows your driver.

THE FIRST RULE OF EQUIPMENT

Any piece of lifesaving equipment will never malfunction or fail until: a) You need it to save a life, or b) The salesman leaves.

THE SECOND RULE OF EQUIPMENT

Interchangeable parts don't, leakproof seals will, and self-starters won't.

THE RULE OF RESPIRATORY ARREST

All patients, for whom mouth-to-mouth resuscitation must be provided, will have just completed a large meal of barbecue and onions, garlic pizza, and pickled herring, which was washed down with at least three cans of beer.

THE FIRST RULE OF BYSTANDERS

Any bystander who offers you help will give you none.

THE SECOND RULE OF BYSTANDERS

Always assume that any physician at the scene of an emergency is a Gynecologist, until proven otherwise.

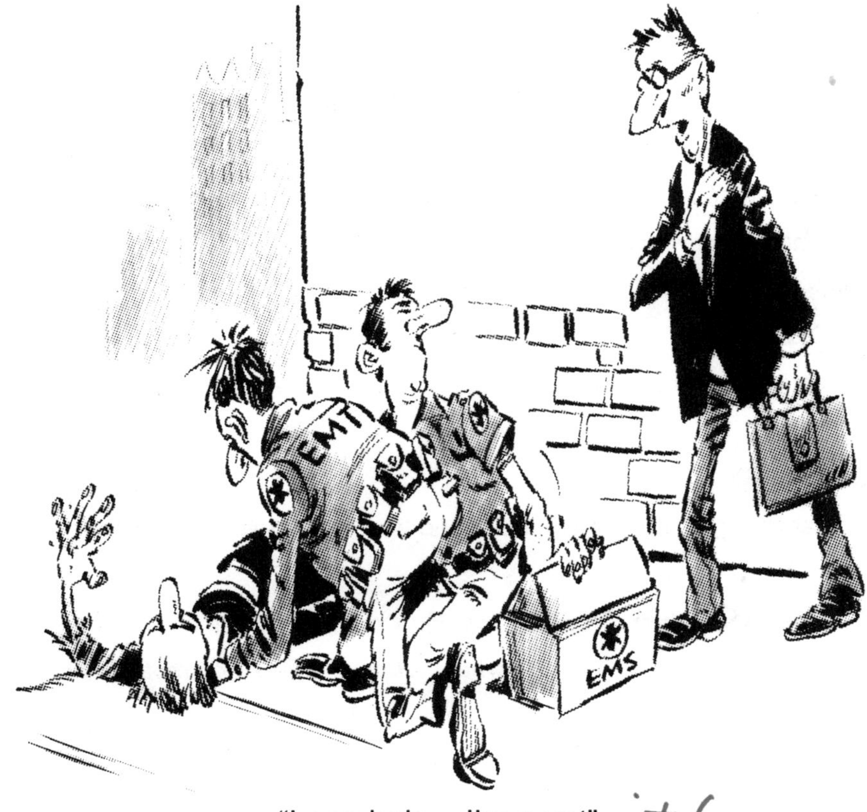

“I can help....I'm a vet” ital

THE RULE OF ROOKIES

1) The true value of any rookie, when expressed numerically, will always be a negative number.

2) The value of this number may be found by simply having the rookie grade his or her ability on a scale from 1 to 10.

For rookie EMTs in the back: 1 = Certified Health Hazard
10 = Member, ACEP,

For rookies driving the vehicle: 1 = Obstruction to Navigation
10 = Mario Andretti.

3) The true value of the rookie is then found by simply negating the rookie's self-assigned value.

THE THEORY OF AMBULANCE INVISIBILITY

Any ambulance, whether it is responding to a call or traveling to a hospital, with lights and siren, will be totally ignored by all motorists, pedestrians, and dogs which may be found in or near the roads along its route.

COROLLARY 1

Ambulance sirens can cause acute and total, but transient, deafness.

COROLLARY 2

Ambulance Lights can cause acute and total, but transient, blindness.

Note: *This Rule does not apply in New York, where all pedestrians and motorists are apparently renderedoblivious to any and all traffic laws.*

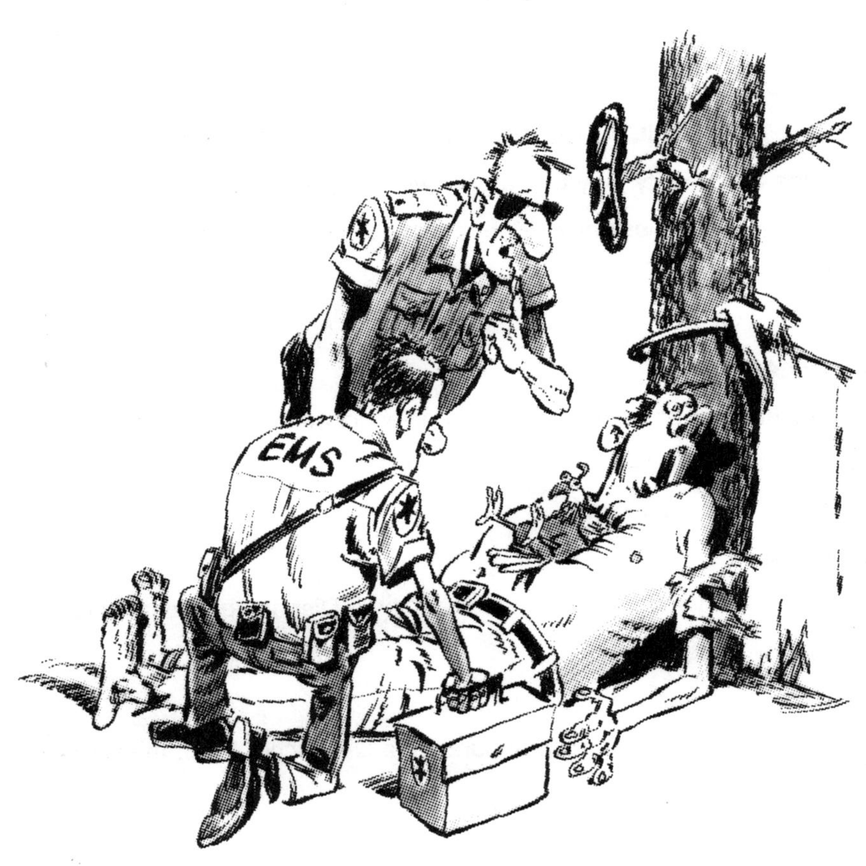

" Quail chest'

THE PARAMEDICAL LAW OF GRAVITY

Any instrument, when dropped, will always come to rest in the least accessible place possible.

THE PARAMEDICAL LAW OF LIGHT

As the seriousness of any given injury increases, the availability of light to examine that injury decreases.

THE BASIC PRINCIPLE FOR DISPATCHERS

Assume that all field personnel are idiots until their actions prove your assumption.

THE BASIC ASSUMPTION ABOUT DISPATCHERS

Given the opportunity, any Dispatcher will be only too happy to tell you where to go, regardless of whether or not (s)he actually knows where that may be.

COROLLARY 1

The existence or nonexistence of any given location is of only minor importance to a Dispatcher.

COROLLARY 2

Any street designated as a "cross-street" by a Dispatcher probably isn't.

COROLLARY 3

If a street name CAN be mispronounced, a Dispatcher WILL misspro-nounce it.

COROLLARY 4

If a street name CANNOT be mispronounced, a Dispatcher WILL mis-pronounce it.

COROLLARY 5

A Dispatcher will always refer to a given location in the most obscure manner as possible. E.g., "Stumpy Brown's Cabbage Field," which is now covered by a strip mall.

THE RULES OF "NO-TRANSPORT"

1. A Life-or-Death situation will immediately be created by driving away from the home of patient whom you have just advised to go to the hospital in a private vehicle.

2. The seriousness of this situation will increase as the date of your trial approaches.

3. By the time your ex-patient reaches the witness stand, the jury will wonder how a patient in such terrible condition could have possibly walked to the door and greeted you with such a large suitcase in each hand.

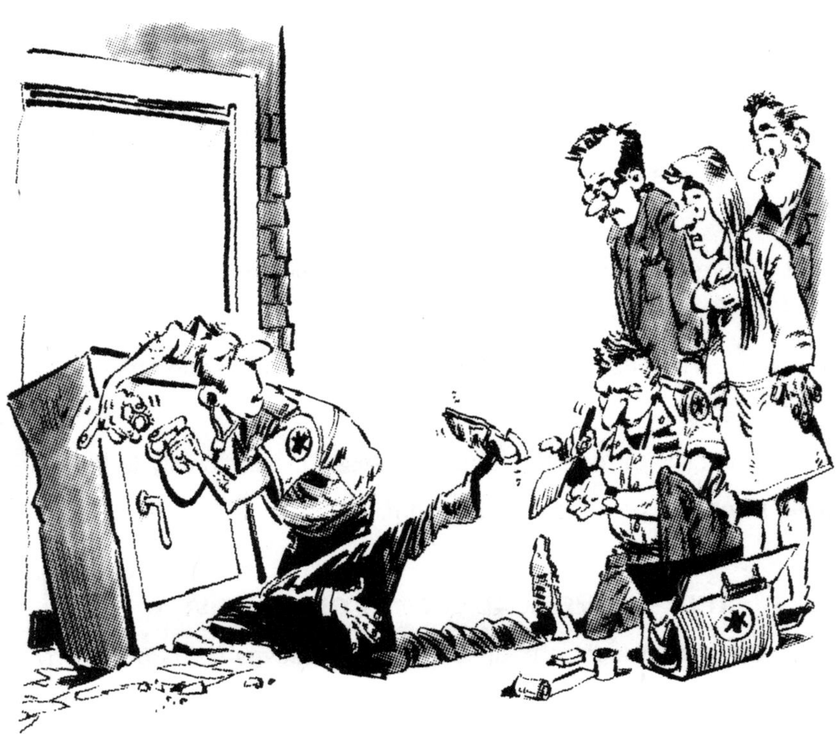

"Vitals! 22 left...16 right" ital

THE LAW OF PROTOCOL DIRECTIVES

The simplest Protocol Directive will be worded in the most obscure and complicated manner possible. Speeds, for example, will be expressed as "Furlongs per Fortnight" and flow rates as "Hogsheads per Hour".

COROLLARY 1

If you don't understand it, it must be intuitively obvious.

COROLLARY 2

If you can understand it, you probably don't.

THE PARAMEDICAL RULES OF THE BATHROOM

1- If a call is received between 0500 and 0700, the location of the call will always be in a bathroom.

2- If you have just gone to the bathroom, no call will be received.

3- If you have not just gone to the bathroom, you will soon regret it.

4- The probability of receiving a run increases proportionally to the time elapsed since last going to the bathroom.

THE PARAMEDICAL THEORY OF RELATIVITY

The number of distraught and uncooperative relatives surrounding any given patient varies exponentially with the seriousness of the patient's illness or injury.

THE PARAMEDICAL LAW OF SPACE

The amount of space which is needed to work on a patient varies inversely with the amount of space which is available to work on that patient.

THE PARAMEDICAL LAWS OF TIME

1. There is absolutely no relationship between the time at which you're supposed to get off shift and the time at which you actually will get off shift.
2. Given the following equation:

T + 1 Minute = Relief Time

T" will always be the time of the last call of your shift. E.g., If you are supposed to get off shift at 1900, your last run will come in at 1859.

THE PARAMEDICAL LAW OF TIME AND DISTANCE

The distance between the scene and hospital increases as the time to shift change decreases.

COROLLARY 1

The shortest distance between the station and the scene is always under construction.

THE PARAMEDICAL THEORY OF TURFING

Any patient who is going to vomit, bleed, urinate, or lose control of their bowels, will be put in the BLS unit.

THE PARAMEDICAL THEORY OF WEIGHT

The weight of the patient that you are about to transport increases by the square of the sum of the number of floors which must be ascended to reach the patient plus the number of floors which must be descended while carrying the patient.

COROLLARY 1
Very heavy patients tend to gravitate toward locations which are furthest from mean sea level.

COROLLARY 2
A patient's weight is directly proportional to the chances the elevator will be non-functioning, and the lights in the stairwell are out

THE PARAMEDIC'S ETOH TEST

Hold your hands about 6 inches apart with thumbs and forefingers touching and ask the patient what color string you are holding. If he indicates a color it is a positive test. Usually corresponds with membership in the 500 Club.

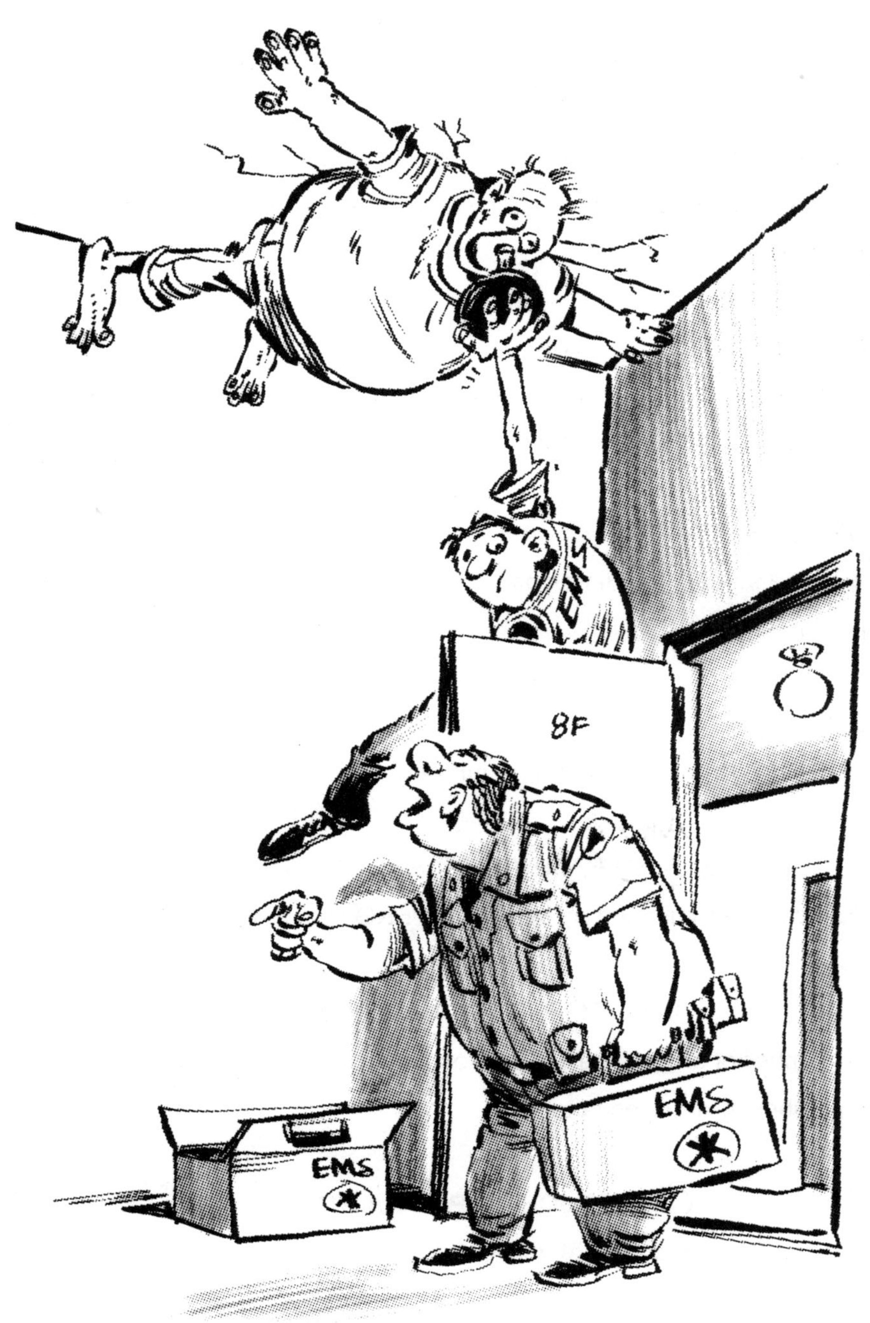

"Damn it Carter, it's not bag, bag, bag, bag, bag,compress.!'

THE LAW OF STATION SHOW-AND-TELL

A virtually infinite number of wide-eyed and inquisitive school-aged children can climb into the back of any ambulance, and, given the opportunity, invariably will.

COROLLARY 1

No emergency run will come in until they are all inside the ambulance and playing with the equipment.

COROLLARY 2

It will take at least four times as long to get them all out as it took to get them in.

COROLLARY 3

A vital piece of equipment will be missing.

DR. AMIN RAMZY'S TELEMETRY THERAPY

PVC's can be eliminated by sending an EKG strip to the hospital.

SPIDER MURPHY'S RULE OF LIFE

The number of drugs a patient has on board is directly proportional to the number of knuckles tattooed.

ST.JOHN'S POSTULATE

When the Captain smiles at you, be very, very afraid.

PITTSBURGH RULE OF THREES

(*As it relates to when cardiac arrests occur*)

Over 300 pounds, under 30 minutes to shift change, over 3 stories up in the building... Remember, DEAD IS DEAD.

THE TRUE TEST OF A PARAMEDIC'S SKILL

The true test of a medic's skill is in their element of surprise. Anyone can work with a fully stocked ALS unit. The real trick is making the patient believe that you can really make a hard copy of the EKG without batteries or administer oxygen without a tank.

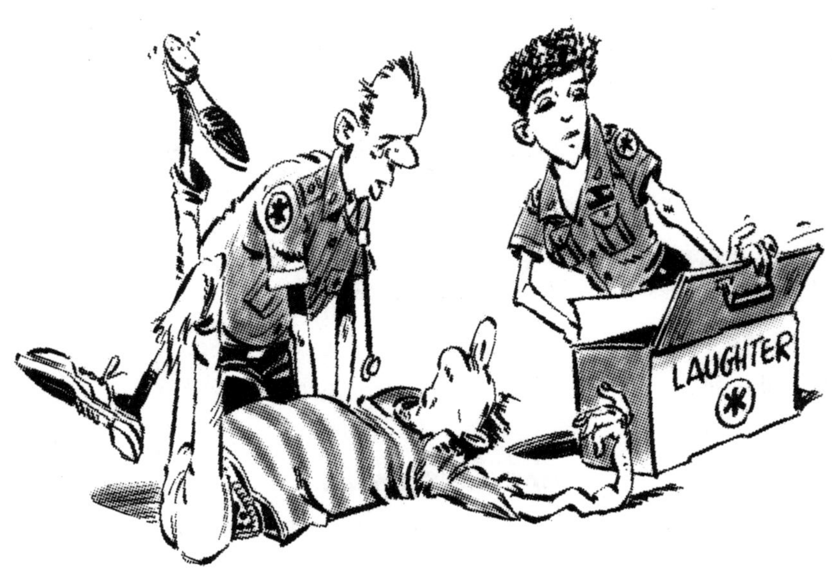

"Sir, were going to give you the best medicine we have"

THE HAZMAT RULES OF PROXIMITY

A HazMat system based on the fact that cops drive right up to vehicles leaking UFL (an unidentified flowing liquid)

1) if the cop is still standing - the scene is non toxic
2) if the paint is still on the cop car - the scene is non-corrosive
3) if the cop car is still running - the scene is not oxygen deficient

THE RULE OF MEETING MANAGEMENT

Mandatory meetings are always scheduled after you've had the night from hell and just want to go home to bed.

THE RULES OF HAZMAT

1. Close one eye. Hold up your thumb. If your thumbnail covers the scene, you're back far enough.

2. If you are pulling up to the scene and the driver runs past you, you are too damn close.

WAYNE'S RULES

1) Patch the holes;
2) Blow the air;
3) Drive the rig.

HAROLD'S MAXIM

Training is learning the rules, experience is learning the exceptions.

Station Watch

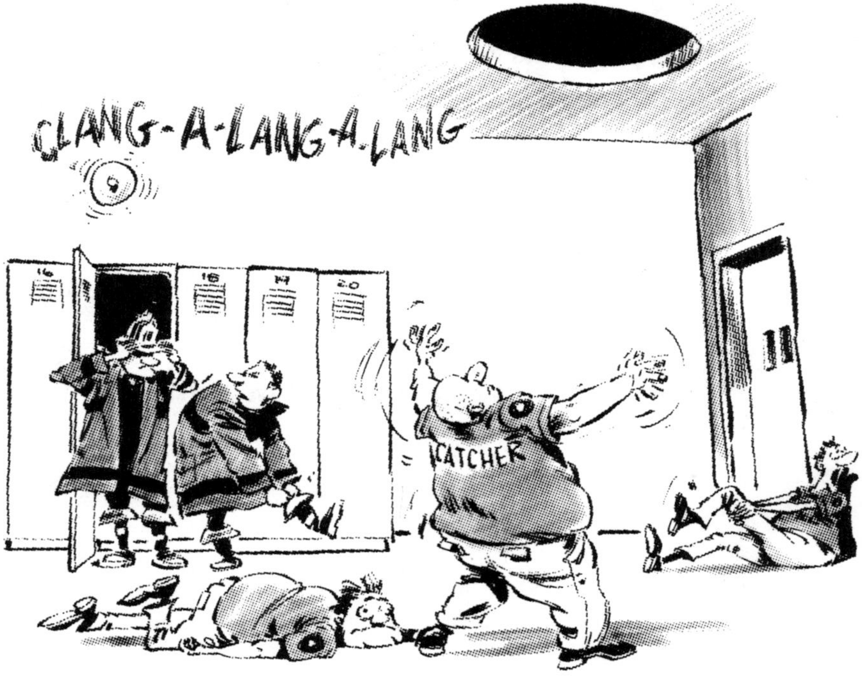

"These damn budget cut's are killing us..!"

Why Fire Engines Are Red

Fire engines are red

Roses are red too

Two plus two equals four

Four times three equals twelve

There are twelve inches in a ruler

Queen Mary was a ruler and also a ship at sea

There are fish in the sea

The fish have fins

The Finns fought the Russians

The Russians are red

Fire engines are red because they are always rushin' ...

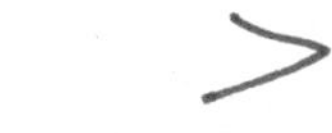

Religious Responders

Last Christmas, while traveling through Georgia, I noticed a community Nativity display that showed the classic scene in great detail. Live sheep and a donkey were included as were all the traditional satues.

One small feature that seemed strange was the fact that the three wise men were wearing fire helmets.

Inquiring at the local fire house, I asked about the helmets.

The Chief immediately looked at my car tags and said "Don't you Yankees ever read the bible?'

I assured him that I did, but that I couldn't recall anything about firemen in the Bible.

He picked up his Bible and thumbed through the pages. Thrusting the book at me he pointed and said" See it says right there that "the three wise men came from afar"

Fire/Rescue/EMS Memorandum
Office of the Chief

To: All Riding Members

From: Chief of Operations

Subject: **Proper Narrative Descriptions**

It has come to our attention from several emergency rooms that many EMS narratives have taken a decidedly creative direction lately. Effective immediately, all members are to refrain from using slang and abbreviations to describe patients, such as the following.

1) Cardiac patients should not be referred to with MUH (messed up heart), PBS (pretty bad shape), PCL (pre-code looking) or HIBGIA (had it before, got it again).

2) Stroke patients are NOT "Charlie Carrots." Nor are rescuers to use CCFCCP (Coo-Coo for Cocoa Puffs) to describe their mental state.

3) Trauma patients are not CATS (cut all to sh*t), FDGB (fall down, go boom), TBC (total body crunch) or "hamburger helper." Similarly, descriptions of a car crash do not have to include phrases like "negative vehicle to vehicle interface" or "terminal deceleration syndrome."

4) HAZMAT teams are highly trained professionals, not "glow worms."

5) Persons with altered mental states as a result of drug use are not considered "pharmaceutically gifted."

6) Gunshot wounds to the head are not "trans-occipital implants."

7) The homeless are not "urban outdoorsmen", nor is endotracheal intubation referred to as a "PVC Challenge".

8) And finally, do not refer to recently deceased persons as being "paws up," ART (assuming room temperature), CC (Cancel Christmas), CTD (circling the drain), or NLPR (no long playing records).

I know you will all join me in respecting the cultural diversity of our patients to include their medical orientations in creating proper narratives and log entries.

How a Plan Becomes Policy

In the Beginning was the Plan.
And then came the Assumptions.
And the Assumptions were without form.

And the Plan was without Substance.
And darkness was upon the face of the Medics.
And the Medics spoke among themselves, saying,
"This is a crock of Shit and it Stinks!"

And the Medics went unto their Lieutenants and said,
"It is a pile of Dung and we can't live with the Smell!"
And the Lieutenants went unto their Captains, saying,
"It is a container of Excrement. It is very strong such that none may abide by it."

And the Captains went unto the Battalion Chiefs, saying,
"It is a vessel of Fertilizer, and none may abide its Strength."
And the BCs spoke among themselves, saying to one another,
"It contains that which aids plant growth, and it is very Strong."

And the BCs went unto the Assistant Chiefs, saying unto them,
"It promotes growth, and it is very Powerful."
And the ACs went to the Fire Chief, saying unto him,

"This new plan will actively promote growth and vigor of the department with powerful effects!"

And the Plan became Policy.

Bennett's Classification for Reading Firefighter Magazines

The Rookie reads entire articles but does not understand what any of it means.

A Firefighter I uses the journal as a pillow during nights on call.

The Firefighter II would like to read article but eats dinner instead.

A Firefighter III skips the articles and only reads the classifieds.

The Master reads and analyzes the entire article in order to pimp the rookies.

The Lieutenant reads the abstracts and quotes the literature liberally.

The Captain reads the entire article, reanalyzes its statistics and looks up all references, usually in lieu of sex.

The Assistant Chief reads the references to see if s/he was cited anywhere.

The Deputy Chief doesn't buy journals in the first place but keeps an eye open for articles that make it into Time or Newsweek.

The Chief reads entire articles but does not understand what any of it means.

Stress Reduction Techniques for Emergency Medical Service Personnel

Here are some ideas to help you through those stressful days...

* Find out what happens to a frog when defibrillated at 360 joules.
* Jam 39 tiny marshmallows up your nose and try to sneeze them out.
* Use your Mastercard to pay your Visa.
* Pop some popcorn without putting the lid on.
* When someone says "Have a nice day", tell them you have other plans.
* Forget the diet center and send yourself a candygram.
* Make a list of things to do that you've already done.
* Dance naked in front of your pets.
* While driving emergency status in the ambulance, tell your partner you're about to have a seizure.
* Put your toddlers clothes on them backwards and send them off to preschool as if nothing was wrong.
* Retaliate to tax woes by filling out your tax forms with Roman Numerals.
* During those late night staging times when your partner is catching a few ZZZZZ's in the passenger seat, slowly move your ambulance into a position right behind a parked semi-trailer, lay on the horn and scream "look out!" (A uniform change for your partner may be necessary.)

* Tape pictures of your field supervisor on watermelons and launch them from high places.
* Leaf through a National Geographic and draw underwear on the natives.
* Pay your electric bill in pennies.
* The next time you're transporting a "frequent" patient, drive to the hospital in reverse.
* Relax by mentally reflecting on your favorite part of the movie* "Mother, Jugs, and Speed" during that important finance meeting.
* Sit right in front of one of your vehicles strobe lights for 10 minutes with your eyelids taped open.
* Polish your ambulance with earwax.
* Start a nasty rumor at your station and see if you recognize it when it comes back to you.
* Bill your doctor for the time spent in their waiting room.
* Lie on your back while eating celery, using your navel as a salt dipper.
* Place an artificial blood capsule in your mouth before approaching your "frequent" patient, then, as if nothing were wrong, let the blood run out while you're asking him questions.
* While on an emergency run, pull up to someone on the sidewalk, makeup a new language and frantically ask for directions.

Top 10...Uh, I Mean 28 Ways to Know if You've Been Watching Too Many "Emergency!" Re-runs. (Fan Version)

* You start dreaming about being rescued by Roy and Johnny.

* You lecture on the dangers of putting your pull tab in the can while still drinking.

* You randomly yell "CLEAR!".

* When driving and weaving in and out of traffic you make airhorn noises, ERRHHH ERRRHHH

* When your voice mail box password is 51564365 (51kmg365)

* You want to name your new born twin sons Johnny and Roy

* When you want to name your new born twin daughters Johnny and Roy!!!!!!!

* You watch a news report of a real rescue which shows paramedics treating an victim and you wonder why they haven't started an IV.

* You watch a news report of a big fire and realise that you're looking for Engine 51.

* When arranging for new license plates for your car, you ask them to check if KMG-365 is already taken......

* You have no medical training yet you can read an EKG.

* You debate the virtues of Boot versus Henry (the station dogs)

* You notice the same stock footage in every episode.

* You use your last stamp to send a fan-mail letter rather than paying your gas bill.

* You have the squad tones as your Window's 95 startup sound file (

* You can't find a particular tape of Emergency! you own because its already in your second VCR

* You start calling people "twit" and "pal".

* You describe the smurfs as cyanotic.

* You recognize "victims" from Emergency! on other TV shows!

* You start your sentences with the word "man".

* You have a special folder for your e-mail labeled "Emergency People".

* You have a special folder in your web browser labeled "Emergency Links".

* You can pick out the misplaced stock footage, due to seeing the old Crown pumper in a scene following a shot of the Ward La France pumper.

* You've scoured the country (and several neighboring countries as well) to complete your collection of episodes no matter how poor the quality of the recordings.

* You can tell which episode it is by just watching the first thirty seconds of the tape.

* You set up a database so you can quickly sort your episodes by tape number, episode number or show title.

* You keep thinking you hear faint sirens even though there's no tape in the VCR.

* You create webpages dedicaed to Johnny and Roy..

How To Tell You'Ve Been Watching Too Many "Emergency!" Re-runs (EMS/FF version)

* You try to convince county dispatch to use the EMERGENCY! tones.

* You use foam on every fire call.

* You are depressed that there isn't an oil refinery in your district.

* When your department orders a new truck and you have it lettered the same as Squad 51

* While teaching a class of new ALS providers about pre-filled syringes, you tell them "Johnny Gage it." (popping the caps off)

* You prefer to use lube and paddles, even though everyone uses remote defibrillators now." (Just so you can rub the paddles together)

* When as a "patient" in a practical exam for EMTs or Paramedics, you list your doctor as Dr. Brackett, and choose to be transported to Rampart.

* You know you've been watching too much Emergency! when you list on the "mark-on board" at your station, Gage and Desoto as crew members on duty!

* When (as a firefighter) climbing into the truck for a call, you climb in, start the truck, and adjust your coat - just like Mike Stoker.

* When pulling out for a call, your officer looks at you and says, "Here we go, Junior.", and you reply, "Ok, Pally."

* When checking your truck, you put the radio transceiver to you ear and say, "Rampart, This is Squad 51..."

* You feel that for any medical problem, from a broken finger to a heart attack, the best remedy is an IV with D5W.

* You're humming the theme song to Emergency! under your breath when responding to a call.

* You get irritated when the sirens for the squad and pumper get reversed in a scene.

* You cringe when they do CPR because you know how to do it correctly.

* “When your station gets a call someone runs over to the station radio and yells “51 10-4 KMG365” :)

* As a firefighter you refer to your station officer as “Cap” — sure the”new kids” do it too, but you are among the few that really know why.

* You mention at an officers’ meeting the idea of putting a “white stripe” on the helmets of captains and lieutenants

* On multi-company responses - -you let the squad lead

* You (try) to wear your helmet in the squad on ALL calls

* You hang your helmet on the hook in the squad — watch your head on that one — OUCH!

* Just after you close the door of the ambulance—you give two good whacks on the rear door

* Instead of “portable” — you refer to the hand radio as “Handi-Talki”

* When firing up the defibrillator — you count out the watt/seconds — even though since the Lifepak”5” they dont work that way anymore

* As a fire dispatcher — you often think, on large assignments (3 engines, 2 trucks and a chief) about adding “Engine/Squad 51” — even if the fire department doesn’t have one

* You dispatch the calls exactly as Sam used to do it, complete with “time out”

Signs Seen in Front of a Firehouse

Several years ago I began changing the sign in from of the firehouse, to display a safety message with some humor so that people would remember it during the day and look forward to the next week's message. Here is a list from the past years.
Chris

You are encouraged to use any of these "quips" that you feel might help get across the important message it contains.
In addition to putting a thought in someones mind you will be reinforcing your community's awareness of the important role of your department.

"Volunteers do it for free!"

"Search & Rescue Officers do it any time, any place, under any conditions and they do it for free."

"Volunteer here! Where else can you have so much fun?"

"Support your local Search and Rescue Squad - Get Lost".

"For a good time, Dial 911- operators are standing by!"

"Our paramedics give you a charge!"

"Hug your kids at home, but belt them in the car!"

"Have you hugged a firefighter today?"

"We brake for your emergency"

"Welcome to (insert your town/city name)- Now, go home safely."

"If you love firefighters - tithe. Anyone can honk."

"Don't laugh. Your daughter may volunteer here."

“Happiness is no one injured at the scene”

“Be safe this weekend. Having a good time can be deadly.”

“Consider yourself hugged”

“If you drink, don’t drive. Don’t even putt.”

“Keep your kids safe. They’ll choose your nursing home.”

“If everything comes your way, you are in the wrong lane.”

“Have another day”

“You light ‘em, we fight ‘em; you crash, we dash.”

“Those who practice safety first, last.”

Safety is no accident.”

“Safety never hurts.”

“Our aim ... no accidents.”

“Safety ... it’s where we want to go today.”

“Safety ... It’s the real thing”.

“Safety is our life line.”

“Safety is a two way street. Look both ways.”

“Live your dream. Volunteer today. Free training.”

“Stay alert! A spill or a slip means a hospital trip.”

“Get smart! Use safety from the start.”

"Safety ... Been there, done that, bought the T-shirt, washed it twice."

"Safety ... Did it, done it, doing it tomorrow."

"Prepare and prevent instead of repair and repent."

"Being safe is like breathing. You never want to stop."

"The light at the end of the tunnel is the headlight of the oncoming fire truck."

"Blocking a firehouse (or fire lane) is a $250 ticket. Don't risk it."

"Be careful. Lose your grip, or an icy slip, gets you a hospital trip."

"Emergencies do not interrupt our work. It is our work."

"Go where the action is. Volunteer. Free training."

"When seconds count, should you be blocking our driveway?"

"Anger is one letter away from Danger. Drive gently."

"A gleekzorp without a ternpee is like a quop without a fertsneet"

"If you can't be good, be careful. If you can't be careful, we'll get a call."

"Don't ruin your day with a DWI or DOA."

"Make a difference - Volunteer here."

"Smoke detectors make good stocking stuffers." (Xmas time sign)

"Think fire safety when decorating this holiday season."

"Practice safe shopping."

"Be the kind of person your dog thinks you are."

"Triumph is just an "umph" ahead of try."

"Santa likes a clean chimney, so do we."

"The earth spins at 1,000 mph. Wear your seat belts."

"Belt your kids in the back seat - away from air bags."

"Safety is an attitude - develop it !!!"

"Forget the hearse - drive safely first.."

"Don't take shortcuts - some injuries never heal."

"Don't lose your head to gain a minute. You'll need your head, your brains are in it! "

"Be safe at work today. Call in sick."

"Don't get paper cuts. They hurt."

"Safety shoes to house your toes; safety glasses on your nose."

"Your wife will spend your 401K if you get killed at work today."

"Work safe! Crushed fingers affect your golf swing."

"Life did not begin by accident. Don't end it as one."

"Unsafe acts will keep you in stitches."

"Get off the car phone. Drive safely without dialing."

"Safety doesn't help you up, it keeps you from falling."

"Accidents hurt — safety doesn't."

"Hearing protection is a sound investment."

“Don’t let the safety net turn into a hearse.”

“The door to safety swings on the hinges of common sense.”

“Forget the hearse with safety first.”

“You may walk on water today, but you’ll stagger on alcohol tomorrow.”

“We came, we saw, we put it out.”

“Kids - Be Safe. If it glows, don’t touch it!”

“If it’s not on fire, it’s a software problem.”

“If you have nothing to do, volunteer here!”

“It’s not the bullet that kills you, it’s the hole. Call 911.”

“Macho does not prove mucho. Do it safely.”

“Put on your seatbelt. We wanna try something.”

“Slower traffic keep right. It that so hard?”

“Trees only hit cars in self-defense. Drive carefully.”

“Veni Vidi Velchro. I came, I saw, I hung around. Volunteer now.”

“Volunteer here. What else can you do at 3 am?”

“You fall, you call, we haul, that’s all.”

“Call 1st, call fast, gotta make that v-fib last, till we shock ‘um, make ‘um jump, get a rhythm, and a pump.”

“Old firefighters never die, they just stop arson around!”

“You flame, we aim”

"Just a Foam call away."

"If you drink and drive, you might as well smoke."

"Put on your seat belt. We want to try something."

"Try something new - seatbelts."

"Heart disease kills more women than all cancers combined. Chest pain? Call 911."

"Belt kids under 12 in back seat away from air bags."

"Green beer and red blood don't mix. Drive safely on St Patricks Day."

"As temperatures rise, stay safety wise."

"Ladder safety has its ups and downs."

"Let's take ladder safety a step at a time."

"Don't use your invention. Think accident prevention."

"Safety takes on a second of your time, but lasts the rest of your life."

"Stretch safety and sometimes it snaps."

"When safety slackens, accidents happen."

"To protect your hands, use your head."

"Those precious fingers, do not ignore, or they could end up on the floor."

"Be careful with your fingers. You need them to pick up your paycheck."

"Look ma' no hands! Wear your gloves."

"When seconds count, should you be blocking our driveway?"

"Trying to make up time? It might cost a life!"

"Walk in the rain, get wet. Work unsafe, get hurt."

"Know safety, no pain. No safety, know pain."

"Work safe, stay alert, your health is precious, dont get hurt."

"1 in 3 people go to the ER each year. Support _VFD."

"National EMS Week May xx-xx. Making a difference - for life."

"Make a difference, volunteer here. Free training. Call XXX-XXXX"

"Put Safety into action — stay out of Traction! "

"Safety never takes a holiday."

"Working safely is like breathing; If you don't, you die!'

"Safety is a state of mind —- accidents are an absence of mind"

"Luck runs out but safety is good for life."

"Better dead sure than sure dead."

"The chance taker is the accident maker."

"A wound neglected may be a wound infected."

"At work at play, let safety lead the way."

"Practice safety in all you do — everyone depends on you!"

“You bet your life when you take a chance.”

“Only fools break safety rules.”

“SAFETY: To be or not to be — there’s no question about it! “

“You can’t get ‘home,’ unless you’re ‘safe.’”

“Alert today - Alive tomorrow.”

“Safety is not automatic, think about it.”

“Leave sooner, drive slower, live longer.”

“Night doubles traffic troubles.”

“Stop accidents before they stop you.”

“Drive as if every child on the street were you own.“

“Better to arrive late than never.”

“Working without safety is a dead end job.”

“Drive with reason this holiday season.”

“Luck runs out, but safety is good for life.”

“Look sharp, don’t get cut.”

“SAFETY! “Behavior for Life”

“Safety, like a good retirement plan, provides for a better tomorrow! “

“Safety” a small investment for a rich future.”

“Why wear safety glasses? If not, you may end up in the dark.”

"A close call reported today, is the accident that does not happen tomorrow."

"Work to be safe, be safe so you can work."

"Health & Safety, words to live by."

"Safety is you."

"Safety is a product we can live by."

"The key to long life is to live safety."

"Safety is something you can not live without."

"Safety makes good dollars and sense."

"Safety is a lifetime achievement."

"If you figit with safety you could lose a digit."

"Safety's intention is accident prevention."

"Safe today - Alive tomorrow."

"Safety's the key to accident free."

"Before you start - Be safety smart."

"Stop! Safety pays."

"Put safety first - Prevent the worst."

"Don't learn safety by accident."

"No injuries to anyone, ever."

"Chance takers are accident makers,"

“Safety ... you do make a difference”

“Safety fits like a glove; Try one on!”

“Safety... you will regret if you forget.”

“Safty is a full time job, don’t make it a part time practice.”

“Safety... It can charm you, or ALARM you!”

“Accidents big or small, avoid them all.”

“What’s it worth - Safety First.”

“10 fingers - 10 toes. If you are not safe. Who knows?”

“Work Safely or hurt greatly.”

“Safety comes before schedule only in the dictionary.”

“Safety isn’t for helping you up, it’s to keep you from falling.“

“The safest RISK is the one you didn’t take.”

“You can profit from safety or recover without it.”

“At work, at home, let safety be known.”

“K.I.S.S. - Keep It Safe and Sound.”

“Make safety a virtual reality.”

“Safe minds and safe actions equal a safe worker and satisfaction.”

“Get in high speed pursuit of safety.”

“Safe actions bring lasting satisfaction.”

"Working safely each day will keep our ambulance away."

"Safetycalifragilisticexpialidocious."

"Eye protection is clearly the right choice."

"Forget the nurse with safety first."

"Be safety smart right from the start."

"Put safety into action - the wishbone will never replace the backbone."

"Safety isn't expensive, its priceless."

"At Work, At Home, Let Safety Be Known."

"30 Days has September. Safety first. Please remember.."

"Safety practices ... do or die."

"Safety ... Do it. Do it right. Do it right now."

"Some have eyes and cannot see. Some have ears and cannot hear, so lets be wise and wear our safety gear."

"Don't learn safety by accident."

"Working safely may get old, but so do those who practice it."

"Safety is as simple as ABC...Always Be Careful ."

"Don't be safety blinded, be safety minded."

"One split second of carelessness could change your entire future."

"Never think working safe is in vain when it could save a life time of pain."

"Turn your attention to accident prevention."

"Your safety gears are between your ears."

"When in doubt, safety wins out."

"Safety comes in cans. I can, you can, we can."

"Don't just preach safety, profit from it."

"Working safely keeps everyone working."

"A "Safety" attitude is one that never hurts to take home with you."

"6" of bruise is better than 6' under - Buckle up! "

"Safety is something you learn from the start, being accident free is doing your part."

"Safety is a frame of mind, so concentrate on it — all the time."

"Before you do it, take time to think through it.."

"Tomorrow - Your reward for working safely today. "

"Know safety - No injury. — No safety - Know injury."

"Safety rules are your best tools."

"Knock out ... accidents."

"Keep safety in mind. It will save your behind."

"Don't be a fool, cause safety is cool, so make that your rule."

"Safety will set you free."

"One safe act can lead to another."

"Keep your eyes on safety."

"Take safety home for the holidays." (a good December slogan)

"Dig in your heels against accidents."

"As temperatures rise, stay safety wise." (a summer slogan)

"Practice Fire Safety. Watch what you heat."

"If you leave accidents behind, don't leave a forwarding address."

"Hearing protection is a sound investment."

"Apply your good intention to accident prevention ."

"Do your work with pride, put safety in every stride."

"Chance takers are accident makers."

"When you gamble with safety ... you bet your life."

"Don't watch her behind. Keep safety in mind! "

"Work Safely and Carry a Big Lunch Box."

"Mine eyes have seen the gory of the coming of the blood, it is pouring down my forearm in a bright red crimson flood."

"Test your smoke detectors. It's sound advice."

"Don't let your house go to blazes."

"Accidents happen within 25 miles of home. Time to move."

"Air bags - Inflation we can live with."

"If you haven't told your family you're an organ donor, you aren't."

"It's not why you cross the road, it's how..."

"You've got to be very careful if you don't know where you are going becausze you might not get there." Yogi Berra

"It ain't the heat, it's the humility." Yogi Berra

"Merry Christmas! Call mom".

"Losing a hand or an arm isn't hard - just operate machinery, and don't use a guard.."

"Be hand-in-glove with safety."

"Get a grip on hand safety. Wear your gloves."

"Speeding? We have two words for you: JAMES DEAN."

"Tailgaters: Is that your hood ornament or are you glad to see me?"

"Tailgating is accident baiting."

"Give unsafe work practices an inch ... They'll take a foot."

"Working without gloves might be macho, but who is going to tie your shoes in the morning?"

"If it seems unsafe .. It probably is!"

"A fall can be a real downer"

"Using gasoline to clean is a fuelish thing to do!"

"Use a ladder improperly and you have nowhere to go but down!"

"Drink OR drive? The choice is yours."

"Unsafe habits can cost you an arm or a leg."

"Only Superman has xray vision. Staying alert is the safe decision."

“Turn off heaters when not in use. Do not make an ash out of yourself.”

“Accidents will happen when the body’s working’ and the mind is nappin’”

“It could be fatal - read the label.”

“Teach your children all the dangers. Poisons can harm as well as strangers.”

“Little Suzy took a drink and no she is no more;
For what she thought was H2O was really H2SO4.”

“The word POISON doesn’t mean a thing to a child.”

“Child safety is an adult responsibility.”

“Big fires start small. Keep little fingers away from matches.”

“Pesticides can kill kids too!”

“A cat has 9 lives with 8 to spare. Your child has but 1 so be safe - beware!”

“Be wise and protect your little tykes, from shocks, burns, and all the likes.”

“Near misses are still accidents.”

“Your neglect can result in his broken neck”

“One for ther road ... One for the ditch.”

“Dont sacrifice your next birthday for a Happy Hour.”

“The designated driver: a friend for life!”

“Dying for a drink? You just might..”

”Dive drunk and you’ll visit prison bars.”

“Think of the people you’ll meet after your car collides on the street.”

"Live electric currents can make dead people"

"Know watts safe! Use electricity wisely."

"Protect your self from the elements. Be careful around stoves."

"Do you have a pair of safety glasses? Why not?"

"The price of not wearing eye protection is outta sight!"

"Its your only pair of eyes. You can always get another pair of safety glasses."

"Eyes are priceless. Eye protection is cheap."

"Where there is smoke, there should be safety."

"One careless flame can burn and maim."

"Don't wait untill you smell smoke. Fire safety is no joke."

"Is a fire extinguisher in your kitchen? Why not?"

"Fires dont start. They are started. Eliminate fire hazards."

"Get alarmed. Use smoke detectors."

"Winter is the flue season. Have your chimney inspected."

"Lit match. Open gas. Explosive fume. Kaboom!"

"Open flame, explosive vapor. Obituary, morning paper"

"Dont wait till you smell smoke. To find out your fire extinguisher is broke."

"Do you have a first aid kit at home?"

"Save a heart. Be CPR smart."

"CPR does not save lives. But people who know CPR do."

"CPR is easy to do. The only person around. May be you!."

"Helping out is always nice. But what a gift to save a life. Learn CPR."

"Know first aid and CPR. But dont forget to call the EMTs."

"Wearing safety shoes. Gives accidents the boot."

"Running shoes are fine for the street. If worn around mowers, you could lose your feet."

"Sneakers may look cool and neat, don't rely on them to protect your feet."

"Its better to be wrapped up in safety than wrapped up in bandages."

"Modern technology does not do away with good old fashioned safety."

"An ounce of safety prevents a whole lot of disaster."

"Accidents leave a lasting impression."

"Can you spare an arm? A foot? A thumb? An eye? Safety spares you the trouble."

"It'll never happen to me won't make a good epitaph."

"Accidents never happen, they are caused."

"Safety is perfection. Win the gold!"

"If you are not working safely you may not be working at all."

"Haste makes waste; take more time, don't lay your life on the line."

"Accidents happen when you hurry."

"Are you gambling with safety or the lives of your family?"

"Keep your frying on the stove. Respect electricity."

"A broken ladder can lead to a bad break."

"Remember accidents don't take vacations."

"When you come right down to it, floors hurt. Work safely."

"Drive with a clear head, and keep it!"

"Sometimes a short cut has more than one meaning."

"Winter driving safety is snow laughing matter."

"Driving takes full attention. Put down the cell phone."

"There are 1000 heart attacks daily. Most have no clues."

"Clot busters work best when given early. Chest pain? Dont wait! Call 911."

"Someone dies in a car crash every 12 minutes. Don't be next."

"If your neighbors house was burning would you want to help? Volunteer today."

"Its good to know what to do. Next time it could be you."

"Dont wait for an emergency to read the warning label."

"Get out. Stay out. Be fire safe."

"Dont make us your designated driver."

"Don't wait until chest pain becomes severe, call 911."

"At the first sign of chest pain, call 911."

"Be aware. Be heart smart. Don't ignore chest pain."

"80% of heart attacks happen at home. Does your family know CPR?"

"Listen to your heart, Chest pain? Don't wait, call 911"

“Heart attacks don’t have to kill. Don’t ignore chest pain.”

“50% of adults don’t know the signs of a heart attack.”

“CPR is for the dead. Know the early warning signs of heart attack. Get help quickly.”

“Teamwork saves lives. Become a part of our team.”

“Drunk drivers take more than chances. They take lives.”

“When you ride your bike, ride with a friend, your helmet..”

“Adults need bike helmets too.”

“Trauma: The number one killer of youth.”

“Designated drivers: Your choice or ours. Please don’t drink & drive.”

“AAA says 4 out of 5 kids are buckled up incorrectly. Are yours?”

“Sparklers are 1500 degrees at the tip.” (4th of July)

“Don’t drive faster than your angel can fly.”

“Drive with Booze, you lose.”

Lights and Sirens

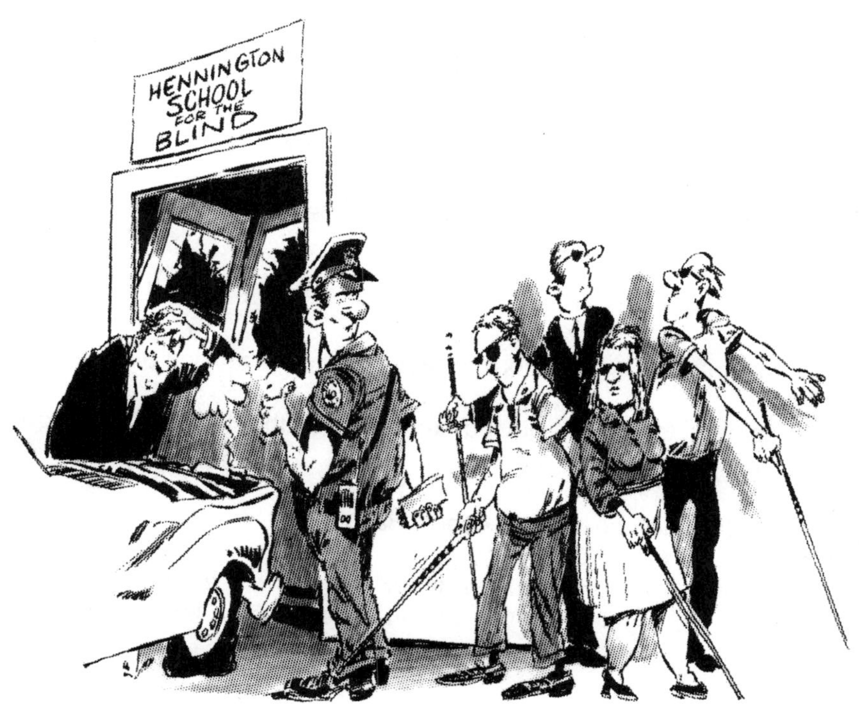

"OK People, move along. There's nothing to see here"

You Might be on a Rural Fire Department if...

1. Your two-way radio procedures all begin with "Breaker Breaker."
2. Your light bar is so scratched up you can't tell when a bulb burns out.
3. You've ever been dispatched on a working "cow" fire.
4. Instead of a Rescue Randy™, your department has a Rescue Bubba.
5. Your department also has a Rescue Cow.
6. You have missed a run before because you were making biscuits.
7. Your aerial ladder keeps getting hung up in all that tobacco hanging from the ceiling of your "station."
8. Your PASS alarm goes "Yeeeeeeee Hah!!"
9. A "controlled-burn" dispatch is actually a code-word for a barbecue that someone is having so you all can get away from the wives for awhile.
10. Dispatch has ever said the phrase "Y'all can't miss it!"
11. Someone asks you the size of your water supply and you respond "Depends on the size of them raindrops."
12. If you flip your badge over, you can see part of a Budweiser logo.
13. You've ever used the high-pressure airbags as furniture around the station.
14. You fill your air bottles at the local gas station's "Free Air" hose.
15. Your parade truck is a flatbed.
16. Your station hot tub is a pickup truck bed with an 1-3/4" stuck in the side and set on fog stream.

17. Your side porch collapses and more than six dogs are killed.

18. There is stuffed possum anywhere in the firehouse.

19, You've ever barbequed Spam on the station grill.

20. The only condiment on the dining table is an economy size bottle of ketchup.

21. The trophy case prominently displays items bought at Graceland.

22. You have more than two members whose name is Bubba or Junior.

23. You think a Volvo is part of a woman's anatomy.

24. You had to remove a toothpick to wear a SCBA.

25. Your idea of a seven course meal is a bucket of KFC and a sixpack.

26. The directions to the station include "turn off the paved road".

27. You have a Hefty bag on the passenger side window of your engine.

28. Redman sends the station a Christmas card.

29. The station bought a VCR so they could tape wrestling while they were on calls.

30. Going to the bathroom in the middle of the night involves putting on a jacket, shoes (if you have them), and grabbing a flashlight.

31. Pork and beans is the gourmet course on the table.

32. You own at least 20 baseball hats.

33. The tobacco chewers at the station aren't just men.

34. Getting a package from the Post Office requires a full tank of gas.

35. Your dress code is: No shirt, no shoes, no problem!

You Might Belong to a Redneck Volunteer Fire Dept if...

1. If your department has ever had two emergency vehicles pulled over for drag racing while going to a scene.

2. If you have naked lady mud-flaps on your pumper.

3. If your firehouse has wheels.

4. If you've ever got back and found you've locked yourself out of the firehouse.

5. If fire training consists of everyone standing around a fire get'n drunk.

6. If you've ever been alerted for an outhouse fire and if that outhouse fire was with an entrapment.

7. If you've ever let a person's house burn down because they would n't let you hunt on their land.

8. If your personal vehicle has more lights on it than your house has lights in it.

9. If you've ever walked through a Christmas display and walked away with at least 3 new ideas for a light scheme for your truck.

10. If your rescue squad can smoke the tires.

11. If your department name is mispelled on your equipment.

12. If the nurses and doctors turn out the lights and hide when you show up at the hospital to get your equipment.

13. If dispatch can't mention your name without laughing.

14. If the local news crew won't put your department on t.v. because you embarassed them last time.

15. If you've ever locked the keys in your trucks

16. If you've ever reffered to a light bar as sexy.

17. If you've ever taken a girl out in a pumper.

18. If your defib consists of a marine battery, a pair of jumper cables, and a fish finder.

19. If your pumper smokes more than the house fire.

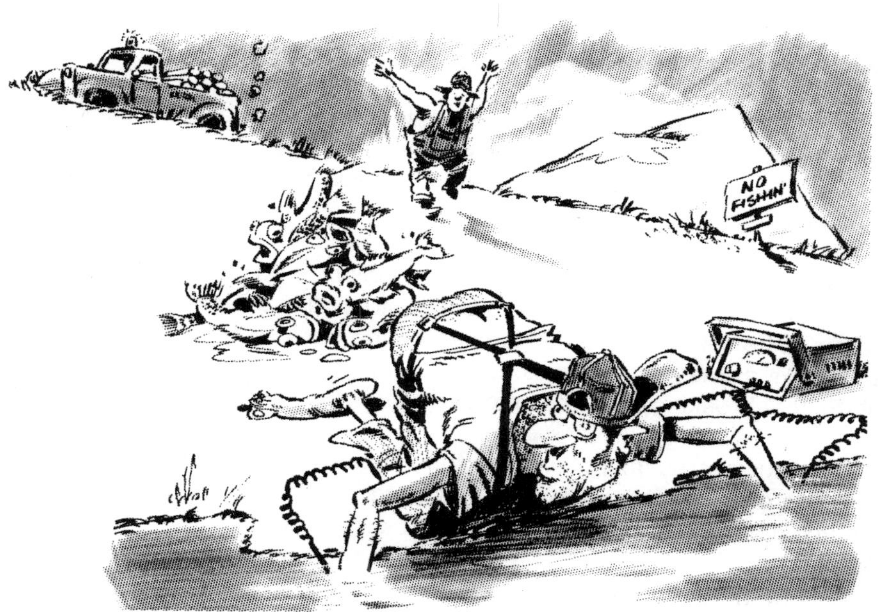

"Leroy, Stop Fishin..the guys need the defib back at the fire hall!"

20. If you've ever been arrested for indescent exsposure at a house fire.

21. If you've ever called it quits on a house fire when the beer got hot.

22. If you've ever been late to a house fire because you had to stop and get the guy who fell off the truck.

23. If you've ever stopped in route to pick up a road kill.

24. If you hand out spit cans before each meeting.

25. If you have a sign out front of your station that says will fight fires for beer.

26. If you're equipment has chew stains down the sides of 'em.

27. If everyone on your department is related in some way or another.

VOLUNTEER FIRE DEPARTMENT

A fire started on some grassland near a farm in Indiana. The fire department from the nearby town was called to put the fire out.

The fire proved to be more than the small town fire department could handle, so someone suggested that a rural volunteer fire department be called. Though there was doubt that they would be of any assistance, the call was made.

The volunteer fire department arrived in a dilapidated old fire truck. They drove straight towards the fire and stopped in the middle of the flames. The volunteer firemen jumped off the truck, and frantically started spraying water in all directions. Soon they had snuffed out the center of the fire, breaking the blaze into two easily controllable parts.

The farmer was so impressed with the volunteer fire department's work and was so grateful that his farm had been spared, that he presented the volunteer fire department with a check for $1000.

A local news reporter asked the volunteer fire captain what the department planned to do with the funds.

"That should be obvious," he responded, "the first thing we're gonna do is get the brakes fixed on that damned fire truck."

You Might be on a Suburban Fire Dept if ...

1. Your pumper carries 1000 gallons of mineral water.
2. Your stress-debriefing program includes an orchestral performance.
3. You take your SCBA home to wear while spraying your lawn.
4. Your department's SCBA has flavored air.
5. Your turnout gear was made by Gucci.
6. Your department's command cars are all red HumVees.
7. You subcontract on the fireground rather than merely call for backup.
8. Your ICS includes a fashion consultant and a hair stylist.
9. Your district's water rescue unit was formerly a yacht.
10. Your deparment's pagers play songs.
11. Your CPR mannequins came from L. L. Bean.
12. Your station has valet parking on runs.
13. Your rehabilitation sector serves caviar and wine.
14. Your department's PASS alarms play classic rock tunes.
15. Your department has a 200 foot aerial ladder but all the structures in the district are 10,000 square foot ranch-style houses.
16. You once missed a run because you broke a nail.
17. You crush aluminum cans for recycling using the Jaws of Life.
18. You've ever taken a call on your cell phone during an interior attack.
19. Your barbecue grill is dirtier than your helmet.
20. There is a bottle of hairspray on each apparatus.

21. Your local disaster plan includes stock market crashes.

22. You've been to an MVA that involved only Rolls-Royces.

23. Your servants ladder the building for you.

24. Training at night requires formal attire.

25. You have no idea what a brush truck is.

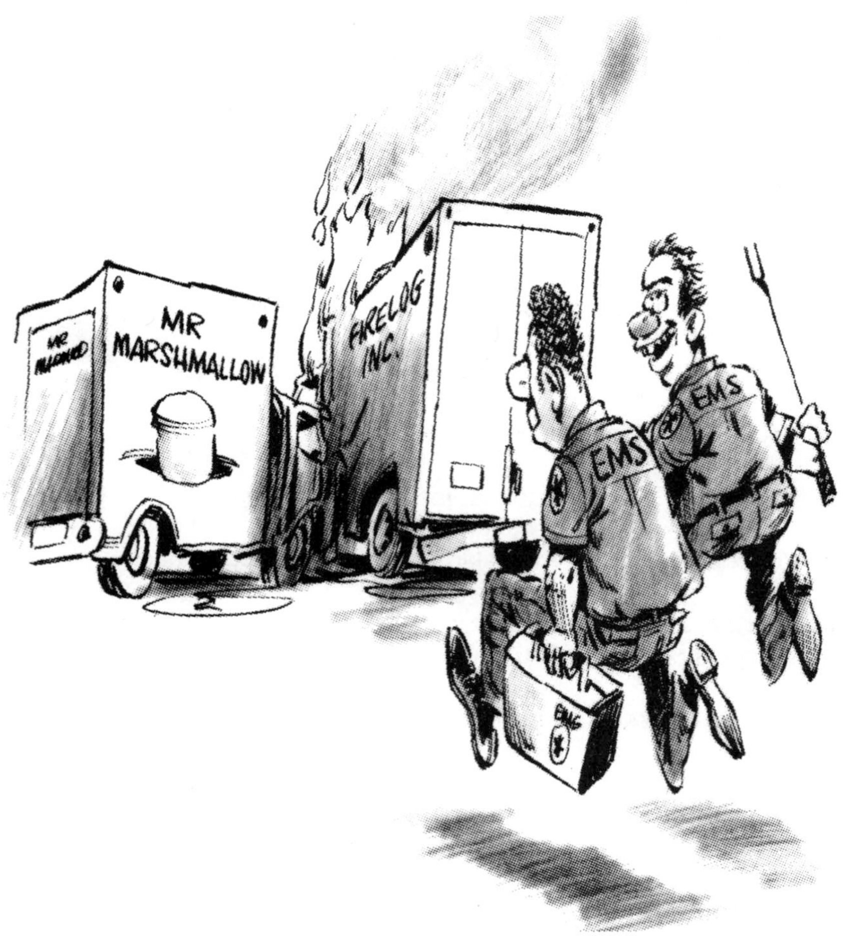

"Man, this kind of thing is the whole reason I joined up!'

On the Fireground

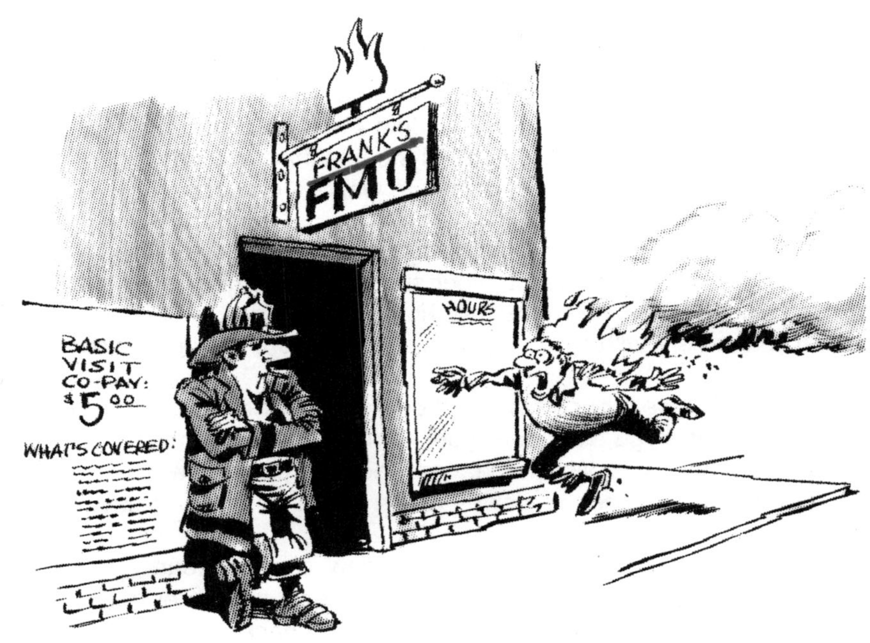

"Where modern firefighting is heading"

A Mexican-American joined a fire dept. He was obviously a really gung-ho firefighter.

When he and his wife had there first child they named him Jose.

When the second one was born, they named him Hose-B.

Brave Volunteers

Scared, cold, in pain, the dust hasn't settled yet.
Pinned in, crying, my clothes are ripped, red, and wet.
Lights, noise, and confusion, all part of the night.
I'm going to die alone, give up the fight.

Red lights are flashing, mixing with blue.
A face appears at my window, the face is you.
"You're gonna be all right" is the first thing you say.
A reassuring voice, someone wants me to stay.

You could have been home with family, they need you too.
You worked all day at the job, your sleeping hours numbered two.
But you went down the hall, hoping your family is OK.
Now you're here with me and Death, with comforting words to say.

No time for yourself, no thought for your safety.
Later you may think, your decision was hasty.
"Get the Jaws. Watch that gas; keep the people away.
Get his vitals, hose this down." Some things I hear them say.

You stand in gas, look in my window, show no fear.
I look back at you knowing, your voice is the last I'll ever hear.
I fade away as you hold me, while holding back your tears.
Thank you for being there, you brave Volunteers.

I Wish You Could

I wish you could see the sadness of a business man as his livelihood goes up in flames or that family returning home, only to find their house and belongings damaged or destroyed.

I wish you could know what it is to search a burning bedroom for trapped children, flames rolling above your head, your palms and knees burning as you crawl, the floor sagging under your weight as the kitchen beneath you burns.

I wish you could comprehend a wife's horror at 3 A.M. as I check her husband of forty years for a pulse and find none. I start CPR anyway, hoping against hope to bring him back, knowing intuitively it is too late. But wanting his wife and family to know everything possible was done.

I wish you could know the unique smell of burning insulation, the taste of soot-filled mucus, the feeling of intense heat through your turnout gear, the sound of flames crackling, and the eeriness of being able to see absolutely nothing in dense smoke—"sensations that I have becomed too familiar with."

I wish you could understand how it feels to go to work in the morning after having spent most of the night, hot and soaking wet at a multiple alarm fire.

I wish you could read my mind as I respond to a building fire, `Is this a false alarm or a working, breathing fire? How is the building constructed? What hazards await me? Is anyone trapped?' or to an EMS call, `What is wrong with the patient? Is it minor or life-threatening? Is the caller really in distress or is he waiting for us with a 2"x4" or a gun?'

I wish you could be in the emergency room as the doctor pronounces dead the beautiful little five-year old girl that I have been trying to save during the past twenty-five minutes, who will never go on her first date or say the words, "I love you Mommy!", again.

(Continued)

I wish you could know the frustration I feel in the cab of the engine, the driver with his foot pressing down hard on the pedal, my arm tugging again and again at the air horn chain, as you fail to yield right-of-way at an intersection or in traffic. When you need us, however, your first comment upon our arrival will be, “It took you forever to get here!”

I wish you could read my thoughts as I help extricate a girl of teenage years from the mangled remains of her automobile, “What if this were my sister, my girlfriend, or a friend? What were her parents’ reactions going to be as they open the door to find a fire officer, hat in hand?”

I wish you could know how it feels to walk in the back door and greet my parents and family, not having the heart to tell them that you nearly did not come home from this last call.

I wish you could feel my hurt as people verbally, and sometimes physically, abuse us or belittle what I do, or as they express their attitudes of, “It will never happen to me.”

I wish you could realize the physical, emotional, and mental drain of missed meals, lost sleep and forgone social activities, in addition to all the tragedy my eyes have viewed.

I wish you could know the self-satisfaction of helping save a life or preserving someone’s property, of being there in times of crisis, or creating order from total chaos.

I wish you could understand what it feels like to have a little boy tugging on your arm and asking, “Is my mommy o.k.?” Not even being able to look in his eyes without tears falling from your own and not knowing what to say. Or to have hold back a long-time friend who watches his buddy having rescue breathing done on him as they take him away in the ambulance. You knowing all along he did not have his seat belt on—sensations that I have become too familiar.

Unless you have lived this kind of life, you will never truly understand or appreciate who I am, what we are, or what our job really means to us.

I WISH YOU COULD!

Murphy's Laws of Firefighting

1) You are not Superman.

2) If it's stupid but works, it's not stupid.

3) When in doubt — Flood it out.

4) Your equipment was made by the lowest bidder.

5) Never share a hoseline with someone braver than you.

6) The important things are always simple.

7) The simple things are always hard.

8) If you are short of everything but smoke, flame and heat, you are in a fire.

9) No pre-fire plan survives the first alarm intact.

10) When you have an area extinguished—dont forget to tell the fire.

11) Anything you can do can get you hurt—including nothing.

12) Radios fail in direct proportion to your need for help.

13) The larger the fire, the less the available water supply.

14) The probability of someone watching you is proportional to the stupidity of your action.

15) Fire is a whole series of circumstances beyound your control.

The Auxilliary

It's been hours for the Company
In hot and heavy gear,
Manning hoses;
Checking pumpers, tankers, motors;
Climbing ladders;
Tearing away debris;
Cutting into twisted metal;
Searching for people;
And pets to rescue;
Or, with the greatest of pain;
And professionalism;
Removing bodies;
Managing traffic;
Checking air packs;
Keeping track of each other;
Saving what they could of the
Precious pieces of people's lives;
And through the sweat and
Soot, heat and exhaustion,
There are those grateful smiles

And quiet thank you's for a simple cup of coffee,

A cold drink, a manwich.

Well done, volunteers -

We'll be back the next time you call us.

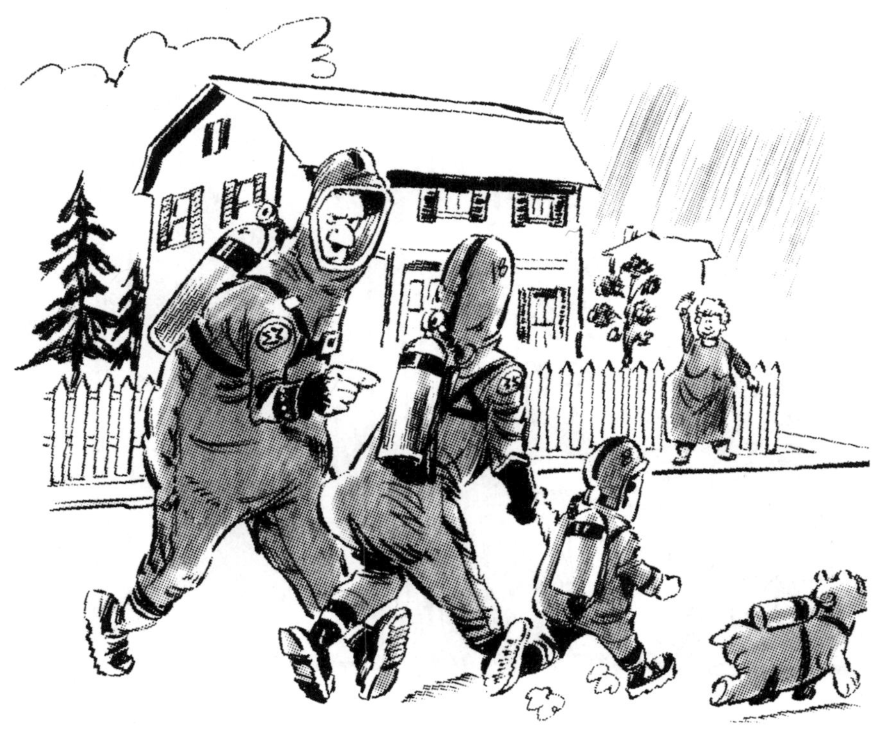

"Sue, I really hate going over for your mother's Sunday Mystery Meal"

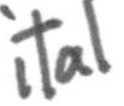

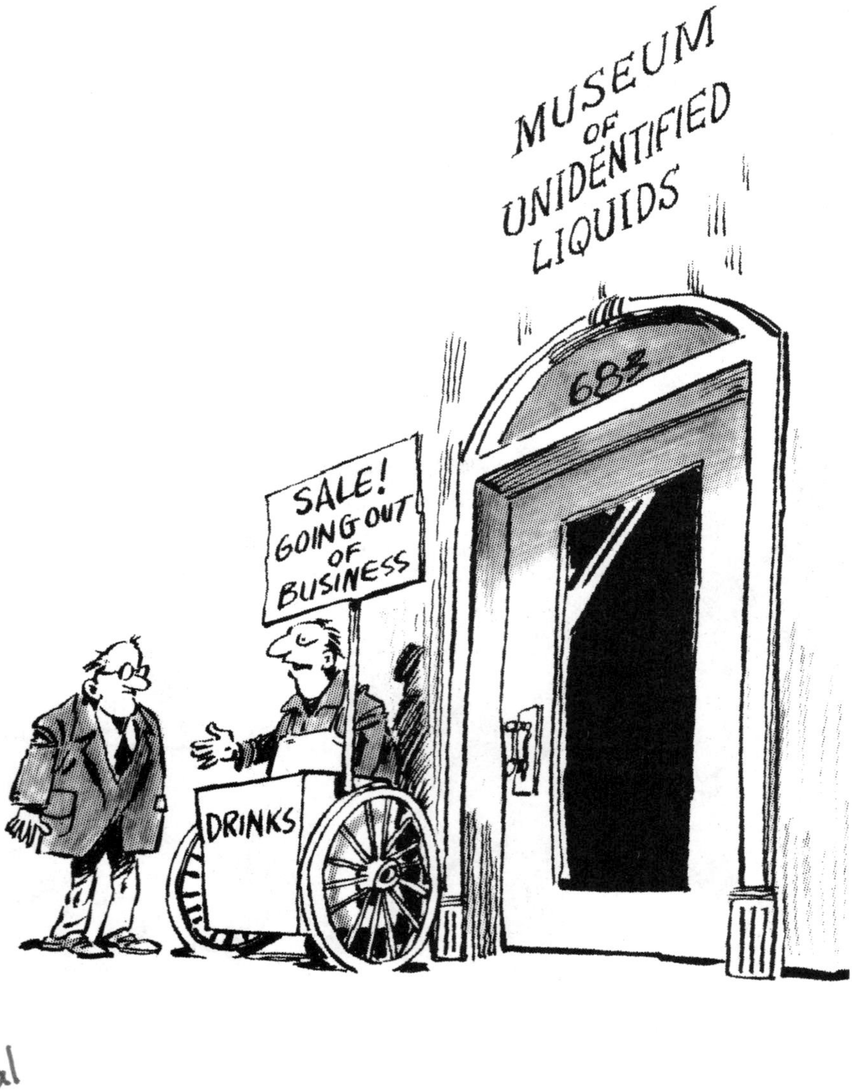

" I Don't Know,..Business has been lousy since I started at this location"

Everything Just Clicks

"Chief, it looks like we got us an organ donor" ital

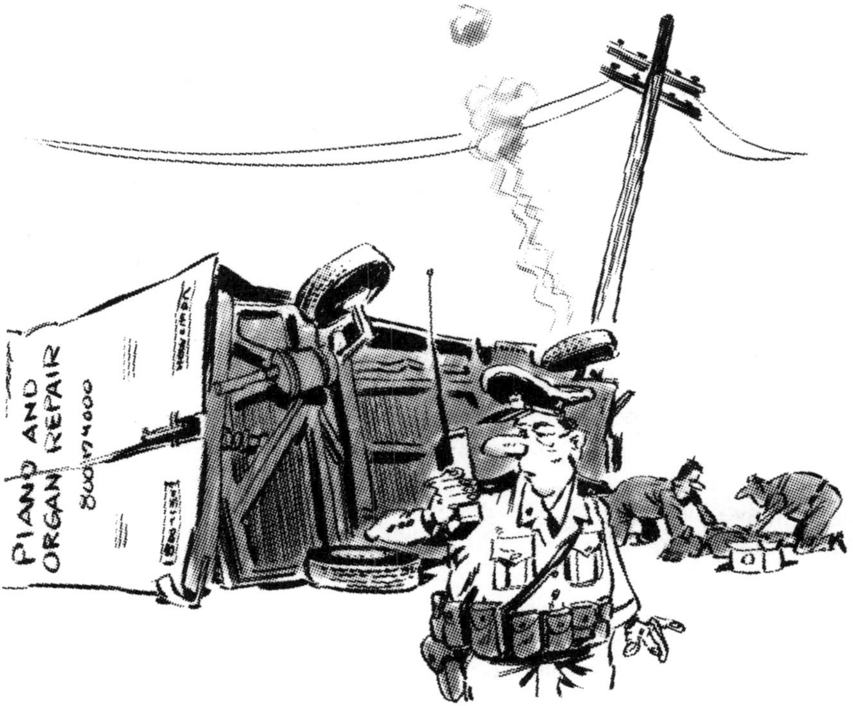

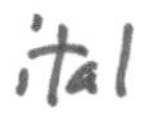

Roadside Oneside

Hello, are you there?
Can you feel my hand on your arm?
Will you talk to me?

Does this hurt?
Please don't move your head,
Do you remember what happened?

Hello, I'm still here,
Can you tell me what happened?
Did you see the other car?

I'm cutting your clothes off.
Did that hurt? Iím sorry.
Show me, show me where.

Shhhh, take a breath for me.
Take it easy now, breath again.
Can you open your eyes for me?

It's just a blanket.
We have to cut the roof off.
Can you feel me touching your legs?

Please, leave the collar on,
What's your name?
Jack? Hi Jack, I'm Jim.

Thatís just the roof coming off.
Dammit Tommy! Please watch the glass!
Sorry Jack, you're really wedged in here.

Jack, now listen.
We're putting a brace on your back.
Please let us do all the work.
I know the straps are tight.
They have to be.

Jack, I'm putting a needle in your arm.
There's still some parts to cut away yet.
Are you with me Jack?
Jack?

Stay with me here, Jack.
No Jack, nobody's gonna die today,
Not on my watch.
Jack, look at me.
Follow my finger.
How many am I holding up?

It's okay Jack.
You can cry.
Yes Jack, you've been badly hurt.

No, everyone else is fine.
They were wearing seatbelts.
No Jack, I wouldn't lie, they're okay.

Please lie still, Jack.
I've got something for the pain,
You'll be going on the helicopter.

Really Jack, look.
I'm smiling.
I don't smile at people who are dying.

Take care Jack,
Get better for that beautiful baby,

I know you'll do it.

St.John's Basic Rules of the Trade

1. Shit happens ...
2. ... Deal with it.
3. Assume nothing.
4. Trust your instincts.
5. Watch your back. Watch your partner's back.
6. Do your ABCs; **A**mbulate **B**efore **C**arry.
7. The mind goes blank as the radio is keyed. Plan for it.
8. At the cardiac arrest, the first procedure is to check your own pulse.
9. If the patient is found in the prone position, something is very, very wrong.
10. A crying child is a good thing; if the child is quiet, be scared.
11. Air goes in and out. Blood goes round and round. Any variation is a bad thing.
12. You can't cure stupid.
13. EMS is long periods of intense boredom, interrupted by occasional moments of sheer terror.
14. Remember your pediatric ABCs: Airway, Airway, Airway!
15. Universal Precautions: If it is wet, sticky and not yours, leave it alone.
16. In emergency care, there are no absolutes.
17. Always answer a Probie's questions, remember what it was like when you were new.
18. Look confident. Look professional.

19. Heaven protects fools and drunks.

20. The rocket scientists that get into car crashes are the first ones to complain how bumpy the ambulance ride is.

21. Turret mounted machine guns would work better than lights and sirens.

22. Paramedics save lives, but it's the EMT skills that save Paramedics.

23. If the patient is sitting up and talking to you, then the patient is not in V-Fib, no matter what the monitor says.

24. It is generally bad to use the words "holy shit" on the scene, in reference to the patients condition.

25. For every 25 calls you run, only 1 will be exciting.

26. Take comfort in the fact that most of your patients survive no matter what you do to them

27. When responding to a call, always remember that your ambulance was built by the lowest bidder.

28. Never let your heart beat faster than the patient's.

29. Always know when to get out of Dodge

30. Always know HOW to get out of Dodge

31. Never go into Dodge without the Marshal

32. There's gonna be paperwork!

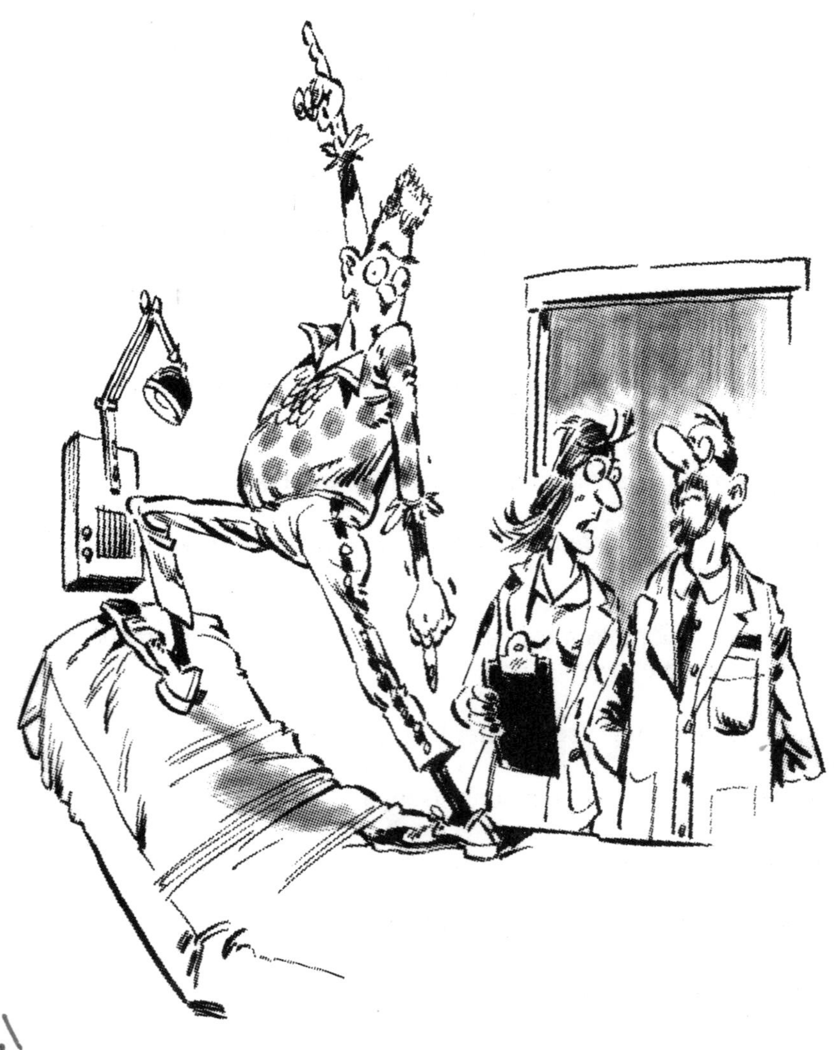

"The medic's that brought him in said they thought it might be Dance Fever."

Communicating in our Unique Language
or
Talk the Talk

Unique Medical Terminology is a necessity brought on by the need to document or chart medical information.This has been adulterated by mixing it with the terminologies used by firefighters. ambulance personnel, police and hospital staff. It has become a common language generally understood by all emergency workers. It also contains key words and phrases commonly heard on the streets.Ethnic references are commonly regional in nature, and may be changed to fit your needs.

Use of these terms will greatly enhance your ability to be able to quickly communicate. This unique language of abbreviations continurs to develop.Should you find any critical terms missing, be sure to let us know.......

We are not sure if this book meets the legal requirements of being a tax deductable purchase, or if your employer will require that you use it as an official reference book.Even if you can't write it off on your taxes, we are sure that you will find it a very valuable assett in expanding and enhancing your abilities to speak and understand the unique language of Emergency Services."

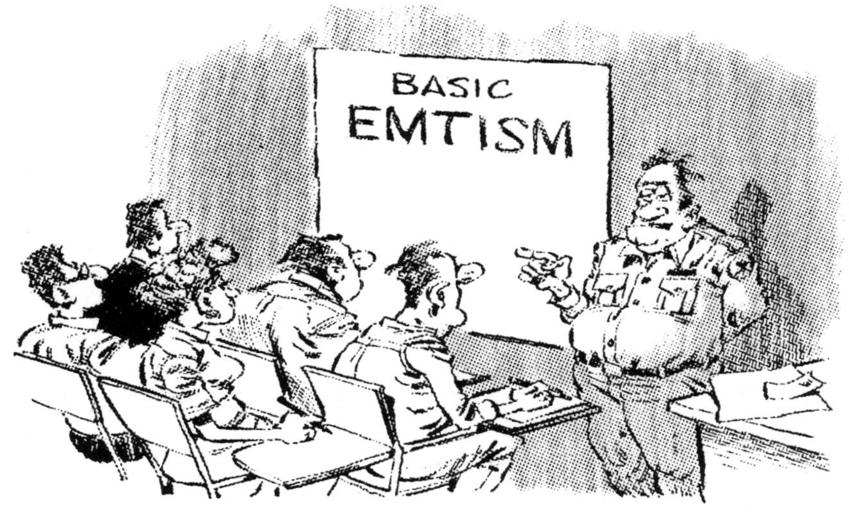

Remember this...the SOB can do a Burnt Worm and end up DRT"

..... **a few of the more common terms we have heard, and used.**

"M" sign	Patient just goes "mmmmmmmmmm"
"O" sign	Patient unconscious with mouth open
"Q" sign	Patient unconscious with mouth open and tongue hanging out
"Dotted Q" sign	A fly lands on the tongue
185 grain Injection	Shot with a 9mm gun
240 grain Injection	Shot with a 44 caliber magnum
4F Club	*Fair, fat, female & forty* - A clue that your abdominal pain patient is a good candidate for cholecystitis (gall bladder disease)
4H Club	*Hemophilia, Hispanic, Homosexual, Heroin abuser* Note: 4H'rs are normally also members of the High 5 Club
500 Club	Blood alcohol >500
ABC	"Ambulance before cops" or "Ambulate before carry" or if you are in a private ambulance company: "Always bill completely"
Abdomen	A shortage of the little Pillsbury guys. (say it slowly)
Achmed	Any middle eastern convenience store clerk
Acid-base	Where junkies hang out
Accordionated	Being able to drive and refold the road map at the same time.

Acoustic	A small length of wood used to coax sounds from certain avians.
Acousticophobia	Fear of accoustics. Common in certain avians.
Acute Angina	Ummm, never mind
Acute Lead Poisoning	Gunshot wound
Acute Thorazine Deficiency	As you might imagine
Adenoma	What you told your mother when you didn't know the answer
ADR	"Ain't doin' right"
Afar	One of those things we put out
Afarmin	Us
Afterbirth	The period of extrauterine life
Afterpains	A period of maternal discomfort following childbirth. Most intense in the offspring's pubertal years.
AGA	"Acute gravity attack" i.e. the patient fell down
AGMI	"Ain't gonna make it"
Agonist	A device or substance that causes extreme pain.
Airborne Ranger	Suicide by fall
Air Conditioned	Multiple GSW
Airway	The three-dimensional space set aside for the flightpath of a jet or plane during takeoff and landing.

Alcohol

A liquid refreshment used by some to "let themselves go" (i.e., to become who they are) and by others to forget who they are. See ETOH

Allstateitis

Neck and back pain developing after an MVA as the drivers exchange insurance cards.

ALS

"Absolute loss of sanity", "Always lifting something", or "Advanced lizard sling-ing"

ALS Units

Super duper pooper scoopers

Ambudexterous

The ability to hold a bag valve mask with two hands while squeezing the bag with your elbow

Ambuslaps

Sharp, double blows delivered to the back door of an ambulance, presum-ably to signal the driver to pull away - often seen on television

Ambusneak

To shut down all emergency lights and sirens several blocks from a scene (see Cloaking Device)

Amp of Holy Water

An irreverent but not calously intended indication that in the failing resuscita-tion effort still underway the next drug to give would be an ampoule of Holy Water as either a miraculous cure or as benediction for afterlife, and as a gentle suggestion that resuscitation efforts be terminated.

AMR

"All medicare recipients"

Anally

Every year

Anaesthesia

A Russian princess you studied in History class

Antacid

Hallucinogenic drugs for little bugs

Anthrax	A trail made by ants
Antibodies	Something uncles are familiar with
Antibody	Your Aunt is Cindy Crawford
APRS	"Acute Puerto Rican syndrome" - bouts of screaming and yelling
AQR	"Ain't quite right"
Arrhythmia	Living an alternative rhythm style
Arson	The guy who Jay Leno replaced
ART	"Assuming room temperature"
Artery	The study of fine paintings
AST	"Assuming seasonal temperature"
Asthma	What to do when Dad says no
Atrophy	A prize for winning the Fireman's parade
Autopsy	Your car hood
BA Bingo	A lottery based on blood alcohol results
Back to 2nd grade	A severe stroke victim
Backdraft	Your pants have a rip in 'em
Bacteria	Behind the cafeteria
Barium	What you do when CPR fails
BATS	"Busted all to sh*t"
Bat Signal	The urgent flailing hand signal from someone who is training a new ambulance driver.

Beltsnarl — Mishandling of an ambulance seat belt by a frantic relative accompanying a patient; typically results in a need for assistance with disentanglement.

Benign — What you be after you be eight

BFC — "Big f*cking crash"

BFL — Big f*cking light" (off the rescue squad)

BFR — "Big f*cking rock" an alternate access device

Bilateral — Someone who speaks two languages

Binky™ Test — The ability of an infant to show basic stability and an interest in "the important things in life" by placidly sucking on a pacifier.

Biologic — Thinking with other parts of your body

Bisexual — A person who pays for sex

Blade — A nickname for a surgeon. (Surgeons are known to be bold and arrogant - often wrong but never in doubt.)

Blaze — A sports coat

BLEVE — "Blast levels everything very effectively"

Blister — A person that shows up after the work i is done.

BLOB — "Bum lying on bench"

Blood Count — Count Dracula

BLS — "Barbaric life support" or "Barely Life Supporting" or "Basic Lifting Service"

BLS Survey — A - Airway, B - Breathing, C - Cancel the Paramedics

Blue Bloater — Description of bodily appearance of COPD patients with Chronic Bronchitis

Bluey on the Green — Cardiac arrest on the golf course

Blurrections - Unintelligible directions from a 911 caller, e.g. "Hang a left where the old schoolhouse used to be..."

BOHICA — "Bend over, here it comes again!"

Botulism — Tendancy to make mistakes

Bowel — A letter like A, E, I, O and U

The Box — Firefighter slang for a modular ambulance, generally called "The Sh*tbox" by those who would rather ride an engine or truck.

Boxed — Put in a pine box (i.e., died)

Brady Brunch — Medication (typically Atropine) administered in an attempt to increase a patient's heart rate.

BRT — "Big Red Trucks"

Breathanol — A gaseous, still-potent form of alcohol found wafting from the mouths of certain EMS frequent fliers

Bronchitis — A dinosaur from the Jurassic Age

Bruise — A six pack of beer

BSS — "Bilateral Samsonite Syndrome" - a patient who is waiting with both their bags packed

BTSOOM — "Beats the sh*t out of me"

Bug Juice — Intravenous antibiotics

Burger's Disease	From eating between runs at too many fast food places
Burn & Return	Radiation treatment patient
The Bus Unloaded	A cluster or "bolus" of patients has arrived in the ER
Patient is BYOB	A drunk
C & A	"Conscious and Alert" as in C&A X3
Cactus Patch	Any fire station full of pricks
Canadian Cruise Missle	Winnebagos
Cancer	Sure I will, Doc.
Canary	A Probie or FNG sent in to see if it's safe. A Blue Canary, in HazMat terms, is a policeman at the scene.
Car vs. pole	"But I only had two beers!"
Cardiac	An old car buff
Cardiac Arrest	Nature's way of telling your patient to take a little dirt nap
Cardiology	The study of poker playing
Cardioplasty	Credit cards
Carditis	Addicted to playing poker
Carpal	People who drive to work together
Castrate	The going price for setting a fracture
Cataract	A whole lot nicer than a Chevrolet
Cathode Ray	The amount Ray billed Cathy
CATS	"Cut all to sh*t"

CAT Scan When the engine crew looks for a lost kitty

Cauterize To make eye contact with an attractive patient

CC "Cancel Christmas"

CCFCCP "Coo-Coo For Cocoa Puffs"

Ceiling Sign The intense physical response including near-levitation from the bed to the ceiling induced by examining for abdominal tenderness in Pelvic Inflammatory Disease.

Charlie Carrot A vegetative patient

Chartomegaly From "chart" referring to the medical record, and "megaly" meaning large or exaggerated in size. Refers to the chart of a patient who comes to the ER very frequently or is a frequent flyer.

CHAOS "Chief has arrived on scene"

"chee-can-breeth" aka Chicken Breath - latino slang for " she can't breath"

Chiaphone When you go to use the phone and it is growing stuff you never learned in biology class.

"Chicken Spray" A nickname used by "oncology kids", for Ethyl Cloride spray, the chilling evaporant liquid used for transiently numbing injection sites.

Choconivorous The tendancy, when eating a chocolate Easter bunny, to bite the head off first.

Chummer A female EMT student who rides along and "chums" for dates.

Civil War Dead Blue on one side, gray on the other.

Clean Jerk What you hope you get when you pick up a body that's been down for a long time.

Cloaking Device A yet-to-be-invented gadget that renders an ambulance invisible to people who have nothing better to do than call 911 instead of a cab.

Closer Someone who can always get the IV in.

Club Med A slow station

Clumfert That invisible extra step at the top and bottom of a staircase. Usually materializes when you are carrying a heavy patient on the stretcher.

CNS-QNS "Central nervous system - quantity not sufficient"

Code Brown A sh*t call

Code Orca A 250 pound+ patient living above the first floor.

Code Surfing Riding the stretcher into the ER while performing CPR

Colic The station sheep dog

Coma A Report punctuation mark

Coma Cocktail 3 medication combinations typically administered for a coma of unknown cause (Narcan, D_{50}W & Thiamine)

Company Social guests

Congenital Friendly

Constipation To have and to hold

Consult w/ Dr Haldol A sedated psychiatric patient

Copulate	Sex between two consenting police offi cers
COPD	"Chronic old persons disease"
CPR	"Cardiopulmonary resuscitation" - the practice of squashing dead people's chests in hopes of squeezing enough blood to the brain to keep them alive for a few minutes more until help arrives. Also called "Cardiac public relations" or "Can't possibly recover" or "Come Put-em-to Rest" or "Check pockets & run" *(from NYC videotape, isn't that a surprise)*
CRAFT	"Can't remember a f*cking thing"
Cranial-Rectal Inversion	Head up their butt
Crash Cart	A form of road accident occuring about the time of Napolean
Crisis Intervention Accessories	Handcuffs and leg irons
Crowning	When you really have to go to the bath-room NOW
CRS	"Can't remember sh*t"
CRT	"Can't really treat"
CTD	"Circling the drain" or "Close to Death" see also FTD
CTS	"Crazier than sh*t"
Cyst	To render aid, as in "Can I cyst you with that ma'm?"
D & C	Where Washington is
Dart 'em	Needle decompression

Dash for Cash — Helicopter transport of critically ill patients. These helicopters are often owned and run by private companies that charge big bucks.

Dash Trash — Paperwork, Burger King wrappers, and other assorted litter that accumulates on the ambulance dashboard

Deceleration Trauma Aggravated by Concrete Poisoning — MVA's into bridge abutments

DDPI — Dead despite paramedic intervention"

Dead Fred in Bed — That early morning "Unconscious, sus pected DOA" call

Death — What some patients do, in the end, to humiliate the paramedic

Deep Fryer — An automatic defibrillator

Defib — Correcting yourself when someone catches you in a lie

Dental — A car after a crash

Depressed — Very sad pants

Dermatologist — A doctor who makes rash decisions.

DFO — "Done fell out" also **DFO-SFJ** "Done fell out - screaming for Jesus"

Diarrhea — The daily station journal

DIB — "Dead in Bed"

Didipee — A question of apparently high importance regarding the patient's history invariably asked by nurses taking a report: colloquial translation of "Did he void? (empty the urinary bladder).

Dilate — To live longer

Diesel Zone — The area to the right rear of an ambulance in high idle at an emergency scene, marked by hot, toxic gases, the atmosphere is inpenetrable by bystanders

DIIK — "Darned if I know"

DILLIGAF — "Do I look like I give a f*ck?"

Dimer — Modern slang, e.g., "These yahoos are a dimer dozen."

DIN — The "Dispatcher is nuts"

DIRTBAG — "Dirty indigent requesting transport because alcohol gives him seizures"

Disconfect — To sterilize the piece of candy you dropped on the floor of the unit by blowing on it, somehow assuming that this will "remove" all the germs.

Dislocation — Dispatcher telling a crew where to go

Ditch Doctors — Paramedics

DMFNFL — "Dumb mother f*cker, not fit to live"

Dockling — The flock of baby interns and students following an attending physician through the corridors of a teaching hospital. (like ducklings lined up behind their mother)

Doing a Burnt Worm — Seizure - aka "Doing the tuna" or "Drop and flop"

Doing the Elvis — Vagal out on the toilet

Doing the Frog — Muscle twitching during defibrillation

Donor Cycles — Motorcycles

Dopamine — Where the Dopas come from

DRT "Dead right there"

DRTTTT "Dead right there, there, there, & there" (Used after train vs pedestrian accidents)

DSB "Drug seeking behavior" - used to describe patients with bogus complaints seeking narcotics in order to dull an otherwise unhappy life.

Duck The portable male urinal - taken from its similar sillouette to the bird of the same name.

Dude Factor A survival scoring factor based on social worth. A **high dude factor** would be an individual of questionable social worth who seems to survive what should be fatal injuries (100+ foot falls, GSW to head/heart, torn aortas from MVA's). A **low or poor dude factor** would be the professional person who slips in the bathroom sustaining a fatal epidural bleed or cervical fracture.

Dump This word has several meanings: 1) When a nursing home dumps a sick patient (usually a negative wallet biopsy) on an ER to be cleaned up and cared for. 2) When a sick patient goes bad, he dumps or crashes.

Dust Farter Beyond elderly

DVR "Darth Vader respirations"

DWPA "Died with paramedic assistance"

Ears Stethescope

Easter Eggs Drinking glasses you find all over the station when you relieve the previous shift.

EKG - FLB	"EKG funny little bumps"
Elderly Mother Trucker	An EMT BLS unit
Electrode	Amount due the electric company
Elixer	What the station dog does to the Chief's wife.
EMD	"Early morning discovery" I.e., he woke up dead.
Emerson Goodwin Sign	When viewing a woman's chest x-ray, a southern doctor may often note: "Emerson Goodwins!"
Emesis	When the patient throws up on his own floor, it's called **EMESIS**. When the patient throws up on the floor of my rig, it's called **VOMIT**. But, when the patient throws up on me, it's definetly called **PUKE**!
EMS Wedgie	The condition of an EMT after being "helped" with a firm grip on the belt accompanied by lifting action, while carrying a patient down a flight of stairs
EMT	"Expensive medicare taxi" or "Every menial task" or "Egg crate mattress technician" "Extra Man on Truck" or "Early morning transporter" or or "Easy moving target" *(from Wash D.C., where else?)*
EMT-I	"Extra man to intubate"
EMT-P	"Expensive medicare taxi provider"
EMTpee	The tentlike structure created by an exhausted EMT pulling the sheets over his head in a vain attempt to get a few minutes sleep

Enema	Not a friend
Engine House	Teepee
ER	The things on yer head that ya hear wit
ETOH	"Extremely Trashed or Hammered"
Exudate	Dating your old lover again
EyeTach	"AYE, YA, YIE, YA, YIE, YA, YIE"
FACBP	"Fellow of the American College of Bystander Physicians" who can easily be indentified at any emergency scene as he shouts orders, typically "hurry up!!!"
Face Plant	Victim falls forward injuring face against floor or other object
Faceprints	Windshield indentations in car crashes
Failure To Fly	The patient fails to achieve the hoped-for discharge criteria and bounces back shortly after discharge; reminiscent of fledgling birds that can't yet leave the nest.
FD	"F*cking drunk"
FDGB	"Fall down, go boom"
Feather Count	A measure of flakiness
Fecal Encephalopathy	Sh*t for brains
Fester	Quicker
FIBD	"Found in bed dead"
FIG-FUBAR	"Found in gutter, f*cked up beyond all recognition"

FIG JAM	"F*ck I'm good, just ask me"
Fibrillate	Tell lies
Fibula	That tiny white lie
FINE	"F*cked up , insecure, neurotic & emo tional"
Fireballs of the Eucharist	Street slang for "fibroids of the uterus"
FIRT	"Failed impact resistance test"

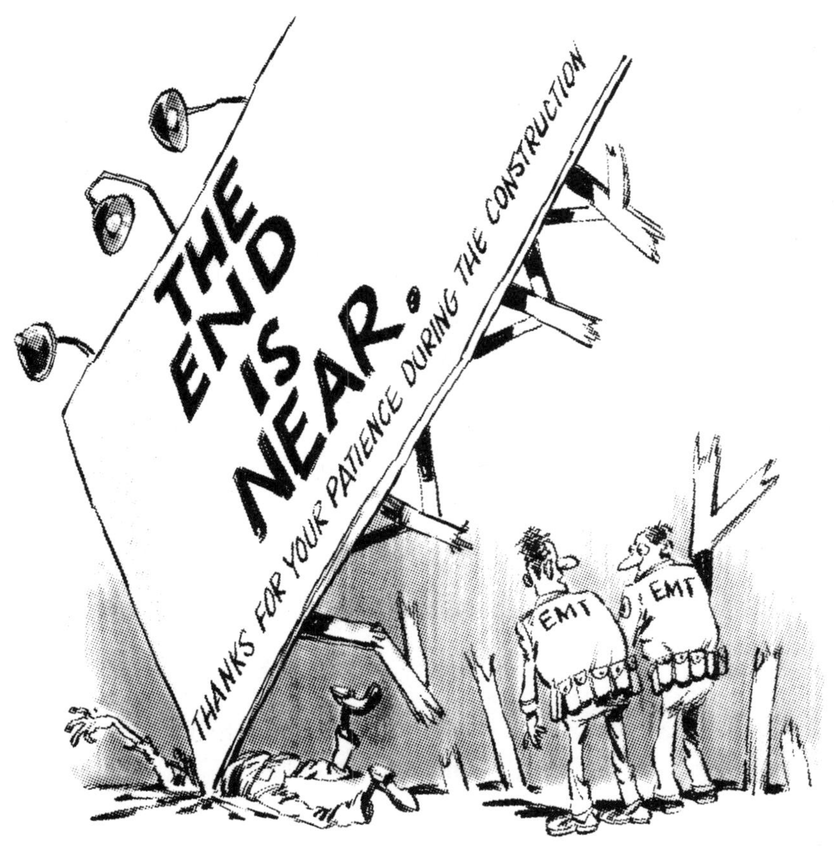

"Is this your first F.I.R.T call?" ital

Fisher-Price	So simple even a fireman couldn't screw it up.
Flares	Flashlight carrying cops who would rather direct traffic than be of any help with the Rescue Techs. **Speed Bumps** are Flares who forgot to replace the batteries in their flashlight.
Flatulate	Fix a tire
FLB	"Funny little bumps" or "Funny little beat" on the EKG
Flea Bites	Phlebitis
FLK-GLM	"Funny looking kid, good looking mom"
Field Flowers	Bloomin' idiots
Fluttering Eye Syndrome	Patient faking having passed out
FNG	Obviously, a "f*cking new guy" or Probie
Foam	Beer head
FOF	"Found on Floor"
Fog Pattern	Diarrhea
FOL	"Full of Liquor"
FOIC	"Fell out in church"
FOOSH	"Fall Onto Outstretched Hand" as a mechanism of injury.
FORD	"Found on road dead"
FOS	"Full of sh*t" i.e., the severely constipated patient with abdomninal pain, or used to describe the patient's story that does not quite hold together.

FOTFL	"Fell on the floor laughing"
FPO	"For practice only"
Fracture	Part of a whole
Freakin' Urination	Frequent urination
Frequent Flyer	They've been on your rig more than three times
Fresh Meat Plant	Fire Training Academy (or EMT school)
FTD	Call the florist, otherwise known as "Fixin' to die"
FTF	"Failure to Fly" aka a botched suicide
FUDD	"F*cked up dead dude" - also called *Elmer FUDD*
Fully Involved	Seriously seeing someone
Fungal	A particularly entertaining female.
Functional Anaerobe	An intelligence impaired individual
Gall Bladder	An anti-Roman vessel
Gangrene	Gang colors on the street
Garage Queen	Any unit that spends more time in the repair shop than on the street.
GARF	Generic term for abrasions, lacerations or contusions in any location, e.g., "He's got one helluva Garf on his head there, Chief."
Gargle	Quasimoto's friend.
Gasper	A patient with sexual asphyxia. Rather, someone who gains sexual arousal by hypoxia during near strangulation.

GD&R	"Grinning, ducking and running"
GDA	"Gonna die anyway"
Genital	Not Jewish
Ghetto Cattle	Pit bulls
Ghetto Pill	Ammonia inhalant
Glovadue	The powder that gets all over your uniform once you've worn your gloves. In contrast to: **Premature Glovulation** - When you get the powder all over your uniform because you put on your gloves and there was no patient to treat.
"Glove up and dig in"	Also known as bowel disimpaction
Glow Worms	HazMat team
GOA	"Gone on arrival"
GoHomey	A transfer from hospital to home
GOK	"God only knows" also used-GORK "God Only Really Knows" (Refers to a puzzling set of symptoms)
Gold Card Patient	A patient who is transported so often, the entire crew knows all the needed info for the chart without asking for it.
GOMA	"Get outta of my ambulance"
GOMER	"Get out of my ER" *(Note:it is commonly believed that GOMERs never die)*
GOMER Tote	The "I don't feel good" call
GPH	"Goddamns per hour"

Gravitational Disassociation	What intoxicated people experience when they fall
Gravity Mediated, Concrete Poisoning	A jumper
GRUNT	"Geriatric retiree unable to navigate traffic" often seen driving Canadian Cruise Missiles
GSH	"Giant sweathog"
GTO	"Gomer tip over"
GTTL	"Gone to the light"
Gut Jockey	A paramedic who rides the engine
H_20	What is on the inside of a fire hydrant. *(As opposed to K_9P on the outside.)*
Haitian Dune Buggy	Car leftovers after the Fire Dept cuts off the doors and roof
Haitian Salute	The patient holding his/her neck after a light property damage MVA
Hamburger Helper	AMTRAK vs pedestrian
Hang a Texaco Drip	Haul butt fast
Hang Nail	A hook for your turnout gear
Haste Cuisine	Your local McDonalds
HazMat UFL	An unidentified flowing liquid
Henway	About 3 pounds
Herpes	What women do in the Ladies Room
HIBGIA	"Had it before, got it again"

High Castor Oil — Elevated Cholesterol levels

High Velocity Lead Poisoning — GSW, aka a gunshot wound

High Five Club — AIDS patient (HIV)

High Rise — When the bread is done

High Serum Porcelain Level — He's a crock

HMO — An actually a variation of the phrase, "Hey, Moe!" Its roots go back to a concept pioneered by Dr Moe Howard, who discovered that a patient could be made to forget about the pain in his foot if he was poked hard enough in the eyes. Modern practice replaces the physical finger poke with hi-tech equivalents such as voice mail and referral slips, but the result remains the same.

Hormone — When the hooker didn't get paid.

Hound Dog & Kojack — Haldol and Prozac

House of Pain — The busiest station in the county/city.

Humerus — Your funny bone

HVLT — "High Velocity Lead Therapy" aka gun shot wound

Hydromatic Breakdance — A swimmer with a seizure or cramps

Hyena Hernia — Hiatal Hernia

Hypertension — A state of nervousness paramedics get while having to start a crying child's IV

Hypodermic — A big fat zoo animal

Hypotension — A state of nervousness medics get when they accidently drop a needle on the floor.

ICU	Peek-a-boo
IDM	"It doesn't matter"
Impotent	A distinguished or well-known patient
Inpatient	Tired of waiting
"Improving His Case"	Victim of a minor MVA or workman's comp injury who wishes and requires no or little other care than documentation of aches and pains for the purpose of a legal claim.
Instant Ambulance	Hip pack carried by a medic
Insurance Pain	Neck pain secondary to a minor MVA
Intern	One after another
Intestine	Taking an exam
IOWA	"Idiots out walkin' around"
ITBNTL	"In the box, nail the lid"
IV	The lady who serves hot chocolate on the Canteen
JAFO	"Just another f*cking observer"
Jerk Juice	Valium
Jesus Bar	The grab bar inside The Box commonly used to hang onto when your driver is overly zealous around corners.
JFN	"Just f*cking nuts"
JIC Tube	A "JIC" blood tube is drawn for "just in case"
Joy Juice	Morphine Sulphate
JP Frog	"Just plain finally ran outta gas"

Juveniles	Little rivers that run into the Nile
Keefart	That moment of time when you slam the locked ambulance door even as your brain says "the keys are in the ignition!"
Kevlodor	The pungent aroma that wafts from body armor after several hours of continuous wear, particularly on a hot day.
Kidney	The joint between a child's hip and ankle
Knife and Forker	A member who only shows up for the social events, also called a "Social Member"
Knockdown	Every boxer's goal
Labor Pains	Getting hurt on the job
Land Tuna	An extremely obese patient
Laser Trace	Asystole (dead as a hammer)
Life Support	Magazine subscription
Lightbar Squirt	The momentary activation of emergency lights as a greeting to passing fire apparatus, police cars, and other ambulances
Line "Em Up	To insert multiple IV lines in order to resuscitate and monitor a critically ill patient
Litter Gitter	The dudes who only schlep gear up and down the stairs
Lizard	Any old person
Lizard Mobile	Any car with a hood too long for a lizard to see over
LMC	"Low marble count"

LOL “Little old lady”

LOL ‘squared’ “Little old lady lying on linoleum”

LOLYNAD “Little old lady in no acute distress”

LPT “Low pain threshold”

MAGGOT “Medically able (to) go get other trans portation”

Magic Juice Cop slang for Narcan

MAP “Mobile anchor point” the largest crew member on the unit

MARPs “Mind Altering Recreational Pharmaceuticals”

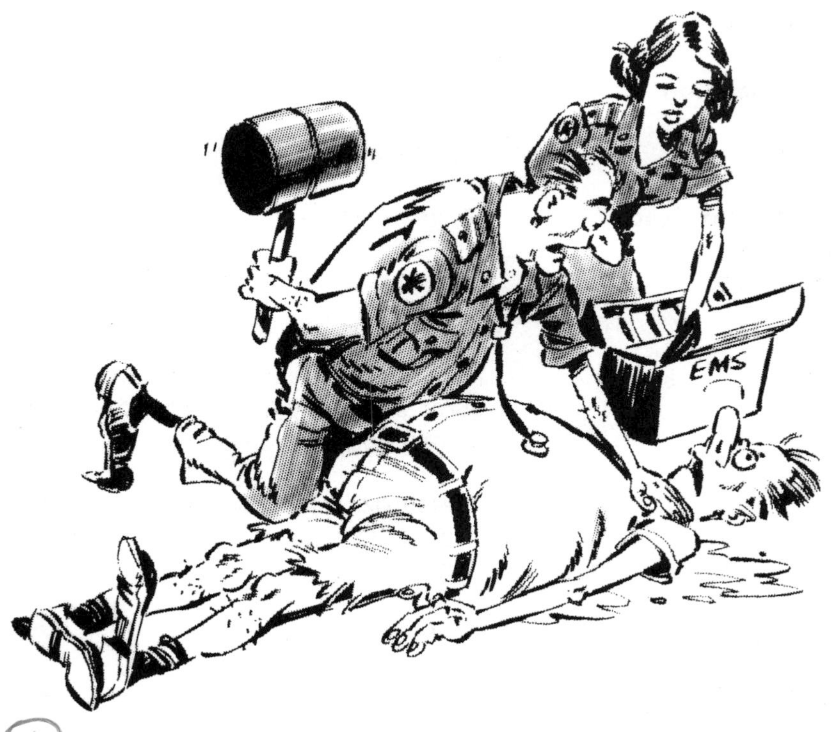

Sorry bout this Sir, but we have just run out of pain killers”

Megahertz — "Oh man, it pains me real bad!"

Medimutes — Patients who have relatives that feel compelled to answer all the questions for them

Metaphysically Challenged — DOA

Metro Valve Prolapse — Must be an urban heart condition

MFAO — "Music for All Occasions" (based on the theory that the right music sets the mood, e.g. Lynyrd Skynyrd's "That Smell" for a MVA)

MGM syndrome — A faker, a person putting on a real good show

Microdeckia — "Micro" meaning small, "deck" as in a deck of cards - hence, a patient playing with less that a full deck.

Minor Operation — Somebody else's

Morbid — A better offer

Mr/Ms Potato Head — A stroke victim

Mr Stay-Puft — A dead body without air conditioning for two weeks

MRB — Maximum resident's benefit (procedures commonly undertaken in the ER to train docklings

MTF — "Metabolizing towards freedom" - (what a drunk does prior to discharge from ER)

MUH — "Messed up heart"

Mutant — A variety of insect that is unable to speak.

MUTT — "Medically urgent, treat and transport"

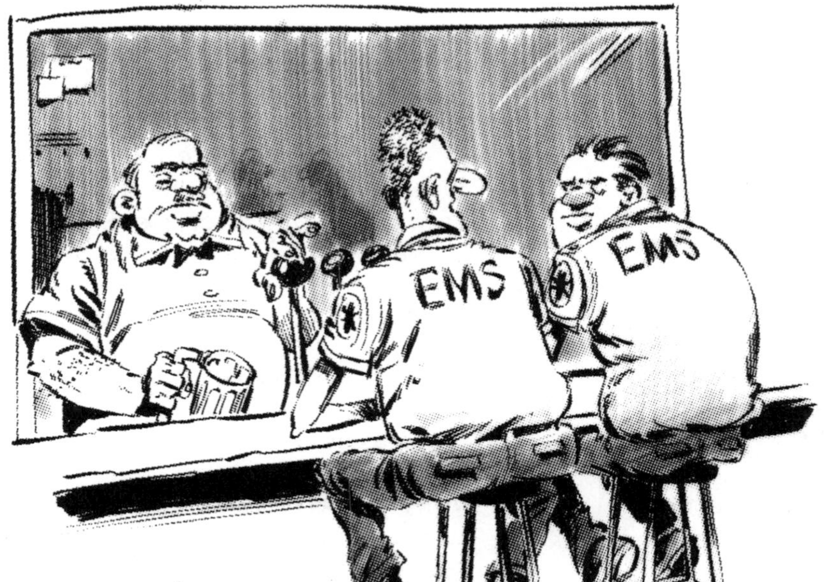

"They fired Thompson today for using something he called his "Sexual Heimlick".

Mycoxafillin — The generic name for Viagra

Nad Noose — When the handle on the foot of the stretcher goes down your pants while lowering it.

NARS — "Not a rocket scientist.

Navigationally Disadvantaged — Your partner cannot read a map

Negative Vehicle to Vehicle Interface — An MVA

Negative Wallet Biopsy — A patient without funds or insurance

Newbee — A person fresh out of training, all full of vim and vinegar

NKDA "Not known, didn't ask"

NLPR "No long playing records (for this guy...)"

Node Was aware of...

Noddy An affectionate term for a night Security Guard or Cop on the midnight shift

Normal Saline When the wind is right, the seas are calm and you are on course. See Saline.

Nose Hose Nasal intubation or nasogastric tube

OB/GYN The "old boy's got ya naked"

OBS "Obvious bullsh*t"

Occular Rectitis When the nerve from your butt to your eyes becomes inflamed and you develop a crappy outlook

ODHG "Overdose of holy ghost" - usual cause of FOIC

Oh Sh*t Call An MVA with a traumatic cardiac arrest or multiple serious injuries

Old Timers Disease Alzheimer's disease

Olfactory Receptor The guy who meets your truck at the loading dock

OLFDGB "Old lady fall down - go boom"

Opsculate To visually measure a patient's vital signs without actually taking them

Ortho Height The elevation of an unattended gurney from which a patient who falls will always get a hip fracture

OTD - DTR — “Out the door and down the road” - aka the patient was finally discharged from the ER

Outpatient — A person who fainted

Outstanding Officer — A company officer who never goes into the building

Paddle User — The person in charge

Palace Guard — Personnel working out of headquarters

PAP Smear — A test for paternity

Parade — The entire station responds (engine, truck, squad, ambulance, and chief)

Paradigm — Twenty cents

Paradox — Two physicians

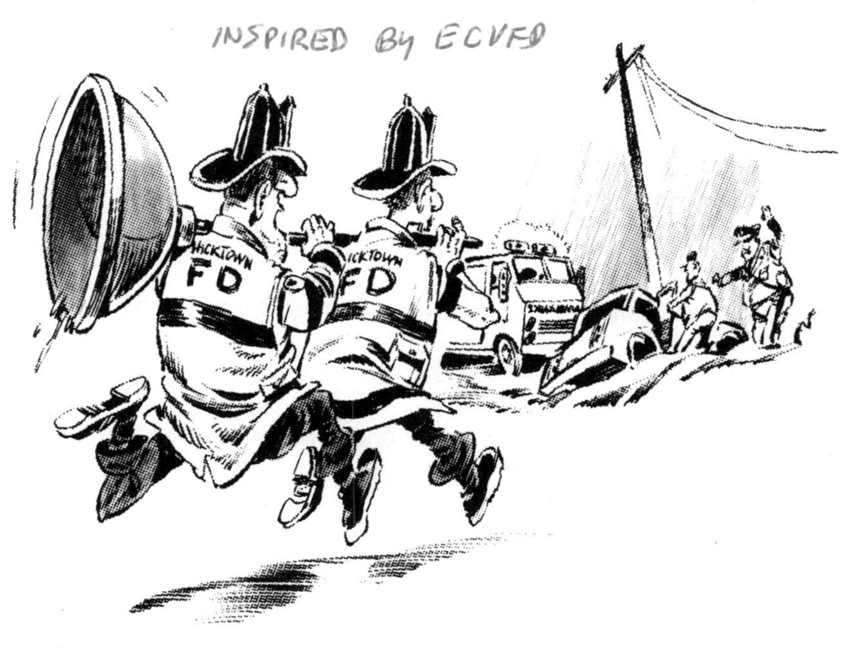

"Quit complaining, the Plunger of Life is all the company can afford".

Para	Just got his paramedic certification and has an attitude
Paralyze	A couple of far-fetched excuses
Para-Pups	Paramedic students
Parasaurus Rex	Any paramedic with over ten years in...
Parasite	Binocular vision
Patella	Grounds for a sexual harrassment case at the stationhouse
Pathological	The best way to get there.
Patient Vu	That strange feeling that you have transported this particular patient before
Paul Alpha	Punitive ALS
Paws Up	Dead
PBAB	"Pine box at bedside"
PBS	"Pretty bad shape"
PCL	"Pre-code look"
PD	"Pretty drunk"
Peanut Butter Balls	Street slang for Phenobarbital
Pelvis	Elvis Presley's cousin
Perch Bait	Body under water for several days
PFO	"Pissed and fell over," aka drunk
PGBFH	"Paragoddess bitch from Hell" or "Paragod Bastard ..."
Pharmaceutically Enhanced Personallity	Cocaine OD

Pharmaceutically Gifted — A steroid user

Pharmanesia — The inability to remember what a patient's medications are for

PHAT — "Pretty Hot and Tempting" (used by either gender)

Phone Book Code — No hope of survival here, so get out the phone book and cross off his name

PIA — "Pain in ass"

PID — "Pink in dere"

Pink Puffer — Description of bodily appearance of COPD patients with Emphysema

Pipe — Any 14 ga or larger needle.

PITA — "Pain in the ass"

Placenta — A Christmas flower

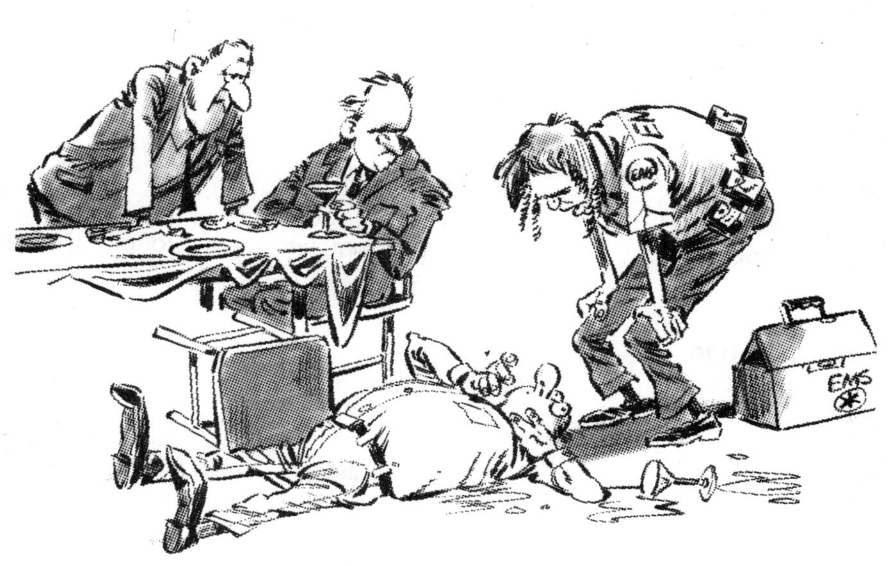

"Hi..My name is Jennifer, I'll be your paramedic for the evening"

Pneumonia — Inventive complaining

PNT — “Paramedic nap

Poke-n-Choke — IV and ET

Polydipose Dysfunction — A big, fat guy

Porcelain Level — A term that stems from porcelain crockery, or a “crock,” as in a “crock of shit”. This is a fictitious blood test ordered in the ER to communicate to a coworker that the patient is malingering and hence a DSB or Terrasphere.

Posh Mortem — Death styles of the rich and famous

PPP — “Piss Poor Perfusion”

Pre-Code — Rapid deterioration or near-extremis, see also FTD

Preictal — A patient who “feels a seizure coming on.”

Probie — The lowest form of life, lower than Whale Sh*t, aka “probationary firefighter”

Prostate — Flat on your back

PUHA — “Pick up - haul ass”

Pull the hook — Tell the Dispatcher to page/tone the vol unteers

PVC Challenge — Intubation

PVL — “Patient - very large”

QID — “Queen in distress” - also known as a “hissy fit”

Quadruple 50 club — 50 years old, PO_2 =50, PCO_2 =50, IQ=50

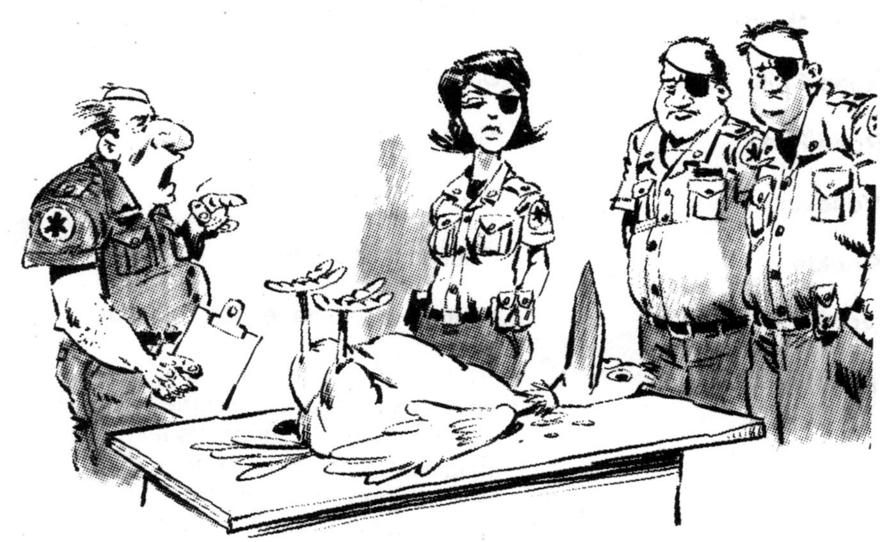

"Let me once again, emphasize ...."extreme caution" on your second attempt at resusci-pet certification."

Raisin Farm — Nursing home

Raisin Hockey — Shuffling nursing home patients back and forth from the ER

Ray — A radiologist - i.e., a person who likes to work in the dark but does not make any decisions. The Radiologist's national flower is the Hedge. (From an ER physician)

RBG — "Received by God"

RBS — "Really bad shape"

Rectum — Damn near killed him!

Rescue Techs — MVA bystanders who take it upon themselves to tell you how to extricate the victim

Rheumatic — Amorous

Ricky Rescue	See "Wacker"
Rigor Morris	The Station Cat is Dead
Road Chili	Unrestrained, ejected, and splattered
Road Pizza	Motorcycle crash victim
Rollover	The station dog's trick
Rookie	Chessboard castle
ROSC	"Return of spontaneous circulation"
RPVU	"Relative Porsche Value Unit" – a surgical index of potential income from the repair of patient injuries, usually orthpedic in nature, e.g., a fractured finger is worth maybe a windshield wiper, a fractured hip – a new set of tires, etc.
S2D2	"Same shit, different day", also (**SSDD**)
Saline	Where you go on your friend's boat
SBOD	"Stupid bitch or bastard on drugs"
Scar	A rolled tobacco leaf
SCENE	"Severe coronary event, not ending"
Scrotal Motor Seizure	Similar to a SF-Scale
Scrotum Scrubber	Hazmat term for a decontamination team member
Secretion	Hiding anything from your sight
"see roaches"	A liver disease often seen in the Hispanic inner city
Seizure	An early Roman emperor

Sex Very short periods of time. Usage:“I’llbe with you in a couple of sex.”

SF Scale Commonly called the Sphincter Factor Scale, e.g., when a car pulls in front of the truck while you are responding to a call. Your SF would probably be a 7 or 8 out of 10.

SFV “S*it for Veins”

S.H.I.T. “Special High Intensity Training”

Shoot and Boot Medicate and discharge

Shock A big fish with sharp teeth

Silver Bracelet Award A special award given to especially disruptive persons by your local police

Singer Technique Rapid and repeated plunging with an IV needle to find a vein, considered very bush league

Siren Silver screen seductress, e.g. Jean Harlow

SOB **Short of breath or Son of (lady dog)**

Social Intubation Deliberate intubation of a verbally abusive patient

Special Assignment Enroute to Mickey-D’s for lunch!

Spooge Sticky residue, usually of an organic origin; generally found on poorly cleaned backboards, laryngoscopes, and other medical equipment, or on ambulance armrests and seats

Spray & Pray What you do when you mess up and take in too small a hoseline.

Squid Any new EMT who can’t wait to get their feet wet.

Squirrels	Overly zealous firefighters (Paid or Vol.)
SRH	"Sperm retention headache"
Stare of Life	The look on the face of a rookie during his first code
Status Asparagus	Vegged out patient
Sterile Solution	Not using the elevator during a fire
Stress in the Firehouse	When you can't find the remote
Successful Delivery	Baby born in the hospital, not in the rig
Suppression	Why you take cough drops
SWAG	"Scientific wild ass guess"
SWW	"Sick, wet and whiny"
Systole	Your sister snitched
T&T Sign	Another survival indicator. If you are toothless and have tattoos, you will survive any insult to your body or its major organ systems.
Tablet	A small table
Tachylordiosis	A patient rapidly screams "Lordy, Lordy, Lordy"
Tachylordy with a Junctional Jesus	"Lordy, Lordy, Lordy, Lordy, Jesus, Lordy, Lordy." This condition usually affects elderly women.
Taking the big bite out of the sh*t sandwich of life	Dying patient. As opposed to "Spitting out a sh*t sandwich" i.e., those who are brought back.
TBC	"Total Body Crunch" The multi-trauma patient

Tape Boogers	Reminants on the patient's skin of old adhesive residue from tape or EKG pads used on a previous call. May be of archeological age.
Tater	A vegged out patient
Tater Toter	Ambulance transporting above
TDS	"Terminal deceleration syndrome" (Usually refers to jumpers and MVA's)
Telexaggeration	An imaginary condition used when calling 911, presumably to make the ambulance arrive more quickly; e.g., "Yeah, he has a broken finger - AND CHEST PAIN.
Terminal Exam	Hint: your last session at the County Morgue
Terminal Illness	Getting sick at the airport
Terrasphere	From the Latin terra, meaning earth, and sphere, meaning ball, i.e. a "dirt-ball".
Test Pilot for Sara Lee	Another fat guy
Throckmorton's Sign	In the unconscious male, the penis points to the injury
Thunderbox	Semi-automatic defibrillator
Tibia	A small country in Africa
TID	"Transient in distress"
Tire Biter	New personnel who haven't passed a Phase 1 exam.
Tissue	Gesundheit!
TLW	"Terrible little wheezer"
TMB	"Too many birthdays"

TNT	"Transport and tolerate"
Touchdown Sign	As you approach the scene, the bystanders are standing on the road-side with both hands in the air.
Toddler Torpedo	Any unrestrained child in a motor vehi cle
Trained Monkey	A medic who follows written protocols without a thought as to what is actually wrong with the patient.
Training	The daily talk shows on TV
Trans-Occipital Implant	A bullet in the head
Trifecta	Flame, death and trauma - all in one perfect shift
TRO	"Time ran out"
Trouser Chili	No explanation needed here
Tumor	An extra pair
Turfing a patient to the BLS crew	Bless 'em, dress 'em & BLS 'em
Two Dude Syndrome	The fight victim who always says "I was minding my own business when these two dudes beat the sh*t out of me"
Urban Outdoorsmen	The homeless
Urinate	What the triage nurse says when she puts you in bed 8.
Urine	The opposite of "you're out"
Varicose **Vein**	Located nearby Conceited
Velcro	The family or friends who came with the patient to the ER in the ambulance.

VIP "Very intoxicated person"

Vitamin V Diazepam

Vitamin H Haldol

VOMIT "Vitals, O_2, monitors, IV, transport"

WADAO "Weak and dizzy all over"

Wailmuffs Secret headgear worn by civilian drivers who don't want to be bothered by the ambulance behind them

Water Hammer Something a Probie is sent to all the stations looking for.

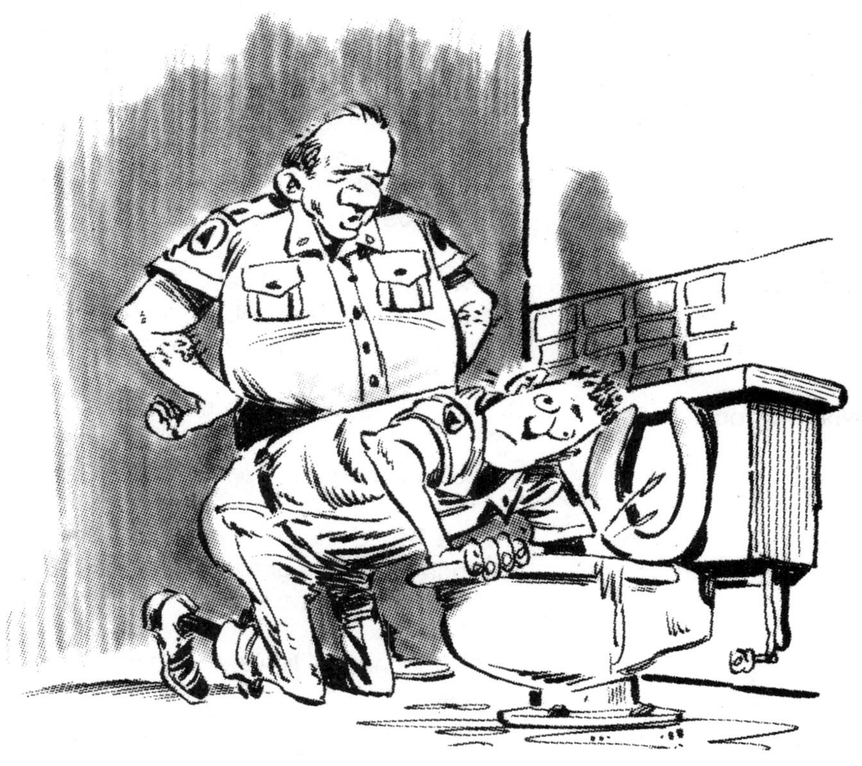

"Check a little deeper...thats where the Captain usually keeps the water hammer." ital

Lower than Whale Sh*t - 1) a recently sworn in Probie
2) **Whale Sh*t** - a Probie with a little more time in.

Wallet Biopsy The only free medical test you will ever see. Usually performed by the hospital insurance department before any patient is treated

Whale Tarp A tarp with handles for carrying 'large' patients.

Weld Defibrillate - as in "I welded him 3 times and he was still in v-fib..."

Whacker The person with 6 emergency lights on their personal vehicle, 7 scanners, 3 pagers, 2 portable radios, and a first aid kit bigger than they are. They are on the Galls Christmas card list. They can't close their dresser drawers because they are too full of T-shirts from big city fire departments they have never been to.

Wheel & Wait Patients who could have driven themselves to the hospital, but instead end up in a wheelchair in the waiting room

Wheel Chock Non-aggressive or worthless personnel

Wiggler Seizure victim

Windmill The frantic relative who has taken it upon himself to gesture as he sees you coming down the street.

WNL "Within normal limits". Often written as a summary for some part of the physical exam, but often sarcastically interpreted as "We never looked."

Woo-Woo A siren

Working-Guy Nod Brief head-twitch of acknowledgement

	from roadside utility workers
WWI	"Walking while intoxicated"
Yahoo	A volunteer who comes out of the woodwork with lights blazing as the house siren and pagers blare. See also <u>Wacker</u>
Yelpkins	Any children who hear your sirens and run out to see the fire truck or ambulance
Yelpswerve	A sudden, violent evasive maneuver performed by a civilian driver who has just realized that an ambulance is behind him
YOYO	"You're on your own"

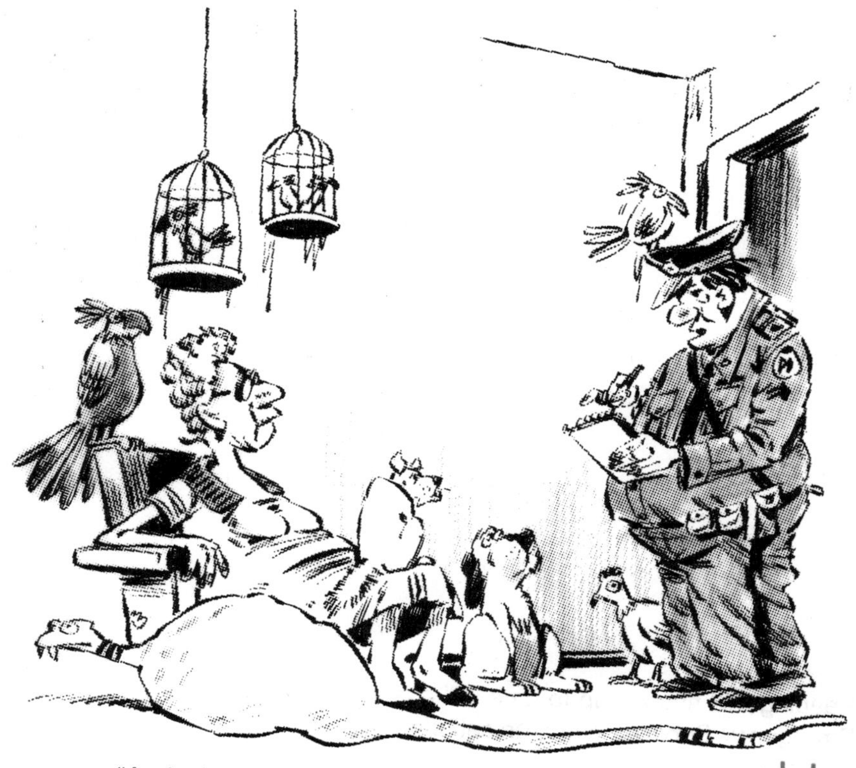

"And when did you last see your husband, ma'am?' ital

Personalized Emergemcy Services "Isms"

This page is provided for you to add you local or personal definitions of those terms critical to your verbal and report writing success.

Due to the constant changes in protocols and procedures as well as the never ending directives that affect your lives, you should strive to continue to upgrade your personal list of "isms"

Keeping this section up to date will assure that you are current in your Emergency Services communications skills.

Doin' Time in the ER

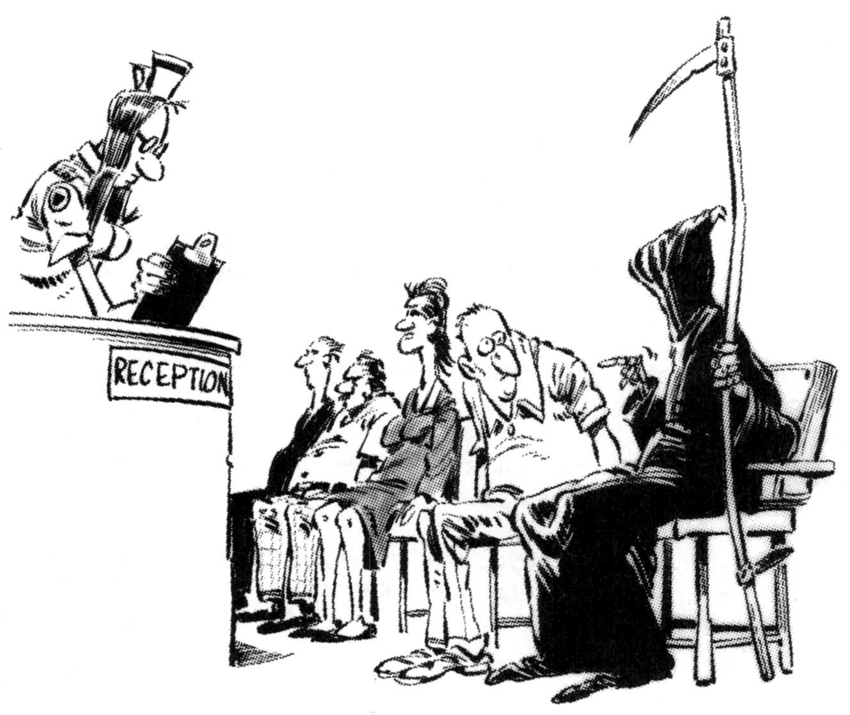

"Yeah...and you think you feel bad."

Note:

This section contains a math for nursing quiz.
(Page 156)

This will be an "Open Book Test"

To assist you, we offer the following hint:

All answers are numbers.

YOU KNOW IT IS GOING TO BE A BAD DAY/NIGHT IN THE ED WHEN:

You show up for work and notice bars have just been installed on all the windows and there is now a metal detector at the hospital entrance.

The paramedics in the parking lot are all using mops to clean up their ambulances and the EMTs are using a hose.

The off-going shift has a hard time keeping a straight face when giving report, especially about Room 15.

Your first patient of the day insists there is no way that she can be pregnant. She's crowning.

Your next five patients and their families all scream at you in different languages, none of which you speak.

Your next patient screams at you in a language you do understand, but you can't remember hearing that many obscenities strung together at once.

The intoxicated 250 kg transvestite in Room 15 keeps trying to get your home phone number because you "are just too sweet."

Your next patient has maggots but isn't dead.

The hospital's attorney wants to talk to you but her secretary won't tell you what it's about.

The hospital has a surprise disaster drill. You were the only one who wasn't tipped off.

The Department is completely empty and one of the off-going shift says, "It's been that way all night, hope you have a quiet day!"

No one remembered to buy coffee.

You have writers' cramp and still have 7 hours of the shift left.

The psychiatric patient who thinks he is Jesus was placed in the same room as another patient who thinks he is Satan.

You get a subpoena for a lawsuit a on a patient that walked out of the department against medical advice two years ago. You can only hope that is what the attorney wants to talk about.

The Hospital Administrator left you a cryptic message about a news crew showing up "sometime today to do a little filming, so everyone act natural."

In the middle of a disaster drill two real trauma patients present themselves.

The paramedics who offered to go out and pick up lunch (and coffee) just advised over the radio they have witnessed a motor vehicle accident involving a transit bus versus a minivan. "Stand by for update."

It's the first day for the new medical interns, paramedic and nursing students all at the same time.

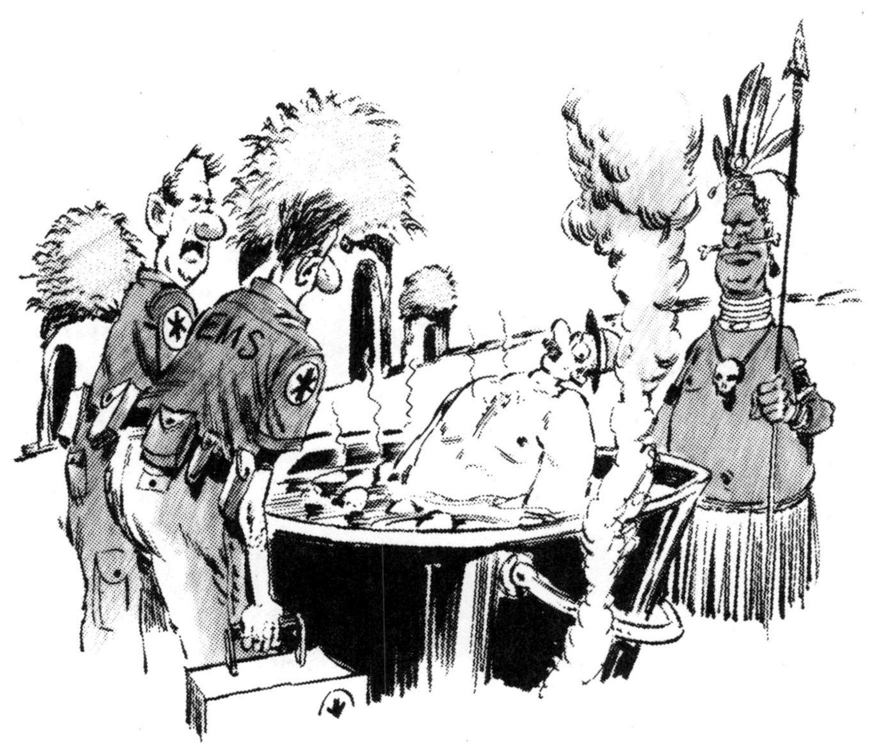

"What do you think?.....another bag of saline and a bag of carrots?"

The paramedics tell you the patient you just received with a closed head injury, flail chest, and positive belly tap is in “much better shape than the one still being cut out of the car wreck.”

You hear there is an influenza epidemic traveling like wild fire through the local nursing homes.

The psychiatric patients’ delusions are beginning to make sense.

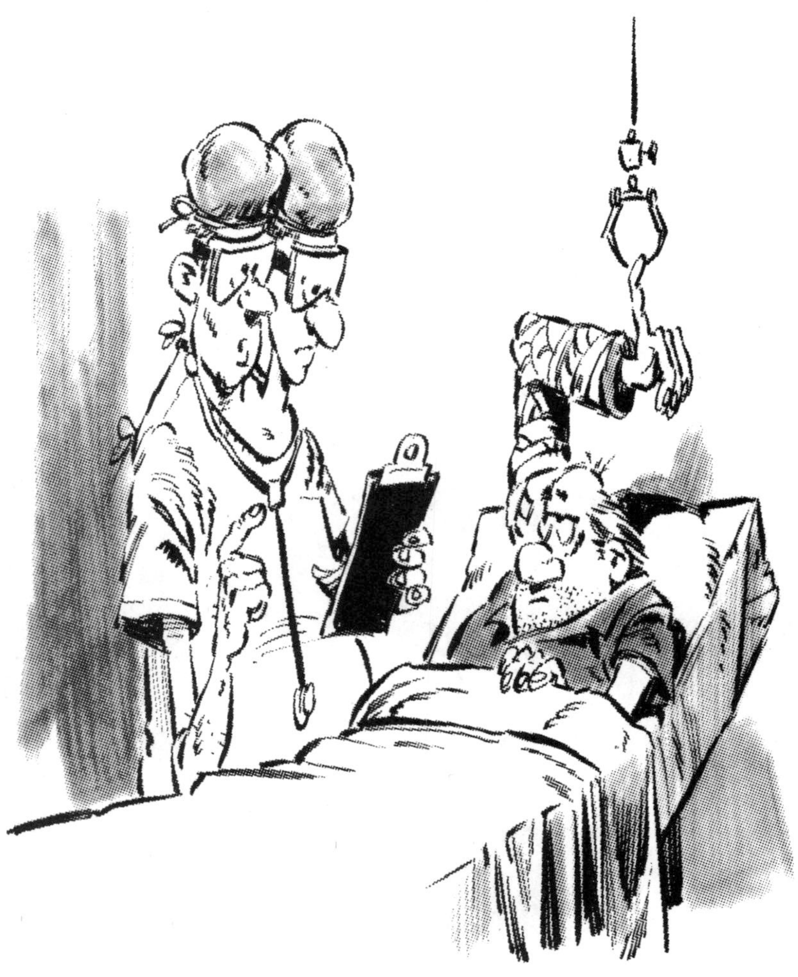

“Now Mr. Wendt, I’ll offer you a second opinion.”

You Might be an E.R. Nurse if ...

You wash your hands before you go to the bathroom.

You have heard patients referring to an ambulance as "my ride"...

You have had a patient start off by telling you what happened at the last three ERs that they went to...

You have ever been told that a stuffy nose at 0300 is an emergency...

You have ever asked, "Why are you here at 3 a.m. if you 've been sick four years?"...

You automatically multiply by two the answer to "How many cigarettes do you smoke per day?"...

You have ever eaten chocolate pudding out of a stool specimen cup, just for laughs...

You have ever wished for a "Dial-a-Dose" Haldol/Ativan tranquilizer gun, and Marlin Perkins to assist you, when sent into the psych room...

You have ever had a patient fail the positive foley test for comas...

You have ever had a patient return to "responsiveness" when the inside of their nose is tickled with a cotton swab...

You know most/all the drunks in town and their case histories...

You can finish a 7 course dinner before anyone else has touched their salad...

You answer the phone "ER" even when you are at home...

You have a pet name for your cardiac monitor...

Your idea of a great dinner is one that's warm...

You know the patient's Medical History better than they do...

You know that all the winos in town give the ER Doc's name when asked who their doctor is...

You know that as long as stupidity remains epidemic in the US, you have job security...

You believe that "ask-a-nurse" is an evil plot thought up by Satan...

You automatically assume the patient is a drug seeker when presented with the complaint of migraine, lower back pain, chronic myalgia (choose one of the above), a list of numerous allergies to meds (except Demerol), and the statement that the family doctor is from out of town...

You don't think a referral to Dr. Kevorkian is inappropriate...

You have ever answered a "lost condom" phone call...

Your idea of a good time is dueling trauma rooms...

You have ever wanted to reply "yes" when someone calls and asks "Is my (husband, wife, mother, brother, friend, etc.) there?"...

You have ever referred to the E.R. Doc or triage nurse as a "shit magnet"...

You have witnessed the charge nurse muttering down the hallway "who's in charge of this mess anyway?"...

You have ever used the phrase "health care reform" to instill fear into your co-workers' hearts...

You believe the waiting room should be equipped with a Valium fountain...

You play poker by betting ectopics on EKG strips...

You want lab to order a "dumb shit profile"...

You are totally astounded when someone from a nursing home is understandable...

You have been exposed to so many x-rays that you consider radiation a form of birth control...

You believe that waiting room time should be proportional to length of time from symptom onset ("you've had the pain for three weeks...well have a seat in the waiting room and we'll get to you in three days")...

You know the phone number to the local Detox Center by heart...

You have ever had a patient control his seizures when offered some food...

You carry your own set of keys to the "leathers"...

Your idea of gambling is an ETOH level pool instead of a football pool...

You have a special shrine in your home to the inventor of Haldol...

Your idea of an x-ray prep is a second dose of Haldol...

Your idea of a CT prep includes Norcuron and a vent...

You have recurring nightmares about being knocked to the floor and run over by a portable x-ray machine...

Your alcoholically challenged patients know you by your first name, and can point to "their room"...

If the hems in your scrub pants are held in with either 3-0 chromic or steristrips...

You've struggled to come up with reimbursable discharge diagnoses such as: acute ambulatory dysfunction, impending asthma attack, constipation (or diarrhea) - resolved, or foreign body in (Fill in the blank) by history...

You've muttered "AMF YoYo" when an obnoxious patient finally leaves AMA (adios my friend - and there is an X rated version to the MF -, but you're on you're own for that one)...

You've ever pretended to sneeze and at the same time thrown KY jelly on a fellow coworker's sleeve in order to make them think that they got shot with a HOCKER...

You've ever sworn that you were going to have "NO CODE" tatooed on your chest (or if you already have it tattooed)...

You have ever tried to hang a "Closed" sign on the ER doors after 0200...

You have ever wanted to print your Discharge Instructions in Comic Book form ...

You recognize the Primary Care Physician for your patients as Dr. None

You have served plenty of GI Cocktails but have never been a bartender...

Your idea of a “Shamrock Shake” has Donnatol and Mylanta in it and doesn’t come from McDonalds...

Your motto is “if its wet, sticky, and not yours, don’t mess with it!”...

You automatically assume that everyone that lists Toradol as an allergy is lying...

You have ever wanted to order a serum porcelain level on all patients that are a crock (or if you have ever asked an intern to order it!) ...

Your favorite drug for combative patients Vitamin H (Haldol)...

You assume every female between 6 and 106 is pregnant until proven otherwise

You feel you look at the world through a proctoscope...

You’ve ever offered your co-worker money to assist with a pelvic exam because you of what you can smell with the patient fully dressed...

You routinely draw a “rainbow” of blood tubes just in case the doctor /resident/intern/student should change his/her mind and order more tests 3 hours later...

You have ever placed a bet on the glucose level of an unresponsive patient (winner is closest without going over)...

You know the phone number of the Coroner’s office by heart... (extra points awarded if you can identify them by voice or badge number)...

You firmly believe that by the time the patient needs the bedpan, they’ve been here too long...

You know the therapeutic advantages of a foley for an unruly patient...

You think “Weed and Feed” refers to IV antibiotics and a NG tube...

Your career highlights include having witnessed the results of 6 or more immaculate conceptions...

You can identify the difference between the PID shuffle and the thorazine shuffle...

Your idea of improved parking lot security includes a "NO FEAR!" window decal...

The last time you saw "management" was in a book...

You include the psych referral people among your best friends...

You plan your summer vacation by the location and reputation of the Trauma Centers...

You can drink a cup of coffee and go straight to bed...

You can define the word "GOMER"...

You've ever discovered that one of your patients is armed by noticing the pistol-shaped image on his pelvis X-ray...

You never (willingly) take a patient's shoes off, no matter what...

Your greatest fear in life involves a pregnant woman shouting "IT'S COMING"...

You don't worry about treating the gunshot wound patient half as much as you do about having to deal with the family (and "visitors")...

You've ever heard someone begin a conversation with "I got this thing stuck in my butt and I can't get it out."...

You realize that effective use of Tylenol, Benadryl and condoms would cut down your work load by 70-80%...

You've ever argued to a drunk that he can't "just walk out" because his leg is broken...

You're on a first-name-basis with all the local street people/bums/homeless...

Your friends and family refuse to watch TV with you if there's a remote possibility that the show will contain any scenes of a hospital (known as the "they're not doing it right" syndrome)...

You can identify the "P.I.D. shuffle" at a distance of 15 feet and the "Kidney Stone squirm" at 20...

You've ever had a patient with a nose ring tell you "I'm afraid of shots"...

You stare at someone in utter disbelief when he or she actually covers his or her mouth when coughing...

You've ever thought "as long as he's got a pulse, I won't worry about that rhythm."...

You think of chocolate, coffee, Coca-Cola and the cafeteria's frozen yogurt when anyone mentions the 4 food groups...

You've ever heard the radio report from the ambulance and put the morgue bag on the cart before the patient arrives...

You think that the announcement of an impending arrival in 5 minutes of two adults in a serious MVA on back boards with sirens on and anxiety a level 10 would be a great opportunity to eat lunch... (and you know that this is more time than you usually get)...

You have ever heard triage nurse first ask, "Is it urgent?" when interrupted from the first break in hours...

You have four categories of patients...urgent, emergent, non-emergent, and S.I.O. (sleeping it off)...

You automatically multiply by 3 the number of drinks they claim to have daily...

You feel that you can diagnose passersby at the mall based on physical presentation...

You don't have to ask "frequent flyers" any medical history questions because you can fill it out from memory...

You can keep a straight face as the patient responds "Just two beers"...

You give the local drunks tips on where to sleep so they (and you) won't be disurbed by a return visit...

You have ever wolfed down a sandwich while emptying your bladder.

You believe that no matter how much you care, some people are just assholes.

When asked, "What color is the patient's diarrhea?", you show them your shoes.

You have more than five pins on your uniform.

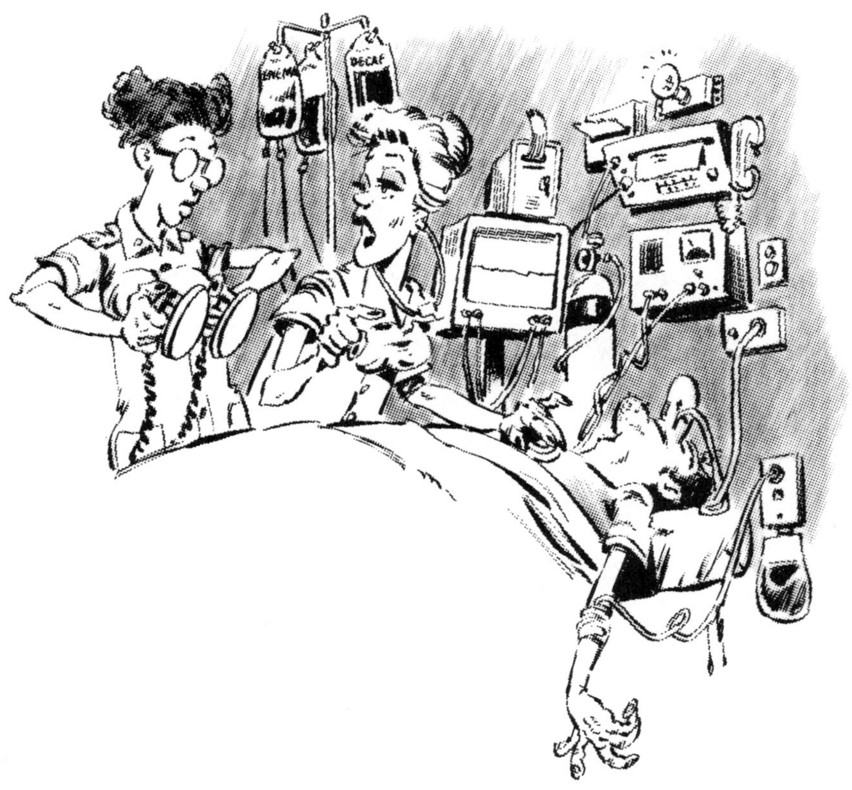

"It's too late !! Someone had him wired to the fax machine by mistake."

ital

Things you don't want to hear from a Trauma Surgeon

1. Better save that. We'll need it for the autopsy.

2. "Accept this sacrifice, O Great Lord of Darkness."

3. Bo! Bo! Come back with that. Bad dog!

4. Wait a minute, if this is his spleen, then what's that?

5. Hand me that? uh? that uh? thingy.

6. Oh no! I just lost my Rolex.

7. Oops! Hey, has anyone ever survived from 500 ml of this stuff before?

8. There go the lights again?

9. "Ya know, there's big money in kidneys? and he's got two of 'em."

10. Everybody stand back! I lost my contact lens!

11. Could you stop that thing from beating; it's throwing my concentra tion off.

12. What's this doing here?

13. I hate it when they're missing stuff in here.

14. That's cool. Now can you make his leg twitch?!

15. Well folks, this will be an experiment for all of us.

16. Sterile schmerile. The floor's clean, right?

17. What do you mean he wasn't in for a sex change?!

18. OK, now take a picture from this angle. This is truly a freak of nature.

19. This patient has already had some kids, am I correct?

20. Nurse, did this patient sign an organ donation card?

21. Don't worry. I think it's sharp enough.

22. What do you mean "You want a divorce"!

23. FIRE! FIRE! Everyone get out!

24. Damn! Page 47 of the manual is missing!

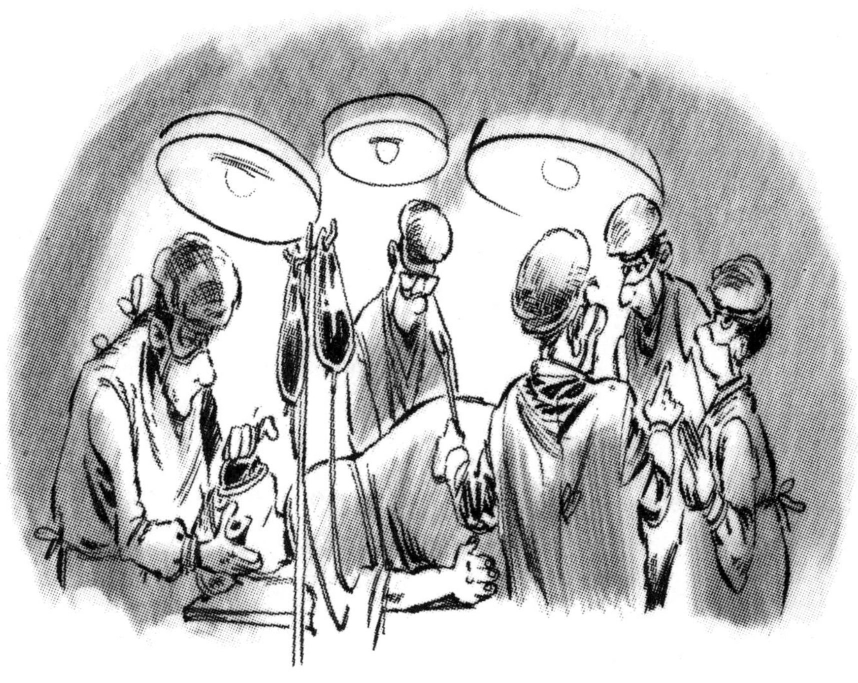

"Nurse Snead, hang one more liter of chicken soup please.." ital

Nursing Rules for the ER

1. Don't hurt yourself.

2. All bleeding stops.

3. Don't lose your cool.

4. Everybody has to die sometime.

5. You can't hurt a dead man.

6. Never yell at other nurses (refer to Rule #1.)

7. Don't get excited about blood loss - unless it's your own.

8. Don't hit patients or doctors - unless necessary.

9. SEX isn't everything, but it's a hell-of-a-long-way ahead of anything that's next.

10. The patient will be alright if he is okay.

11. The pain will go away when it stops hurting.

12. Do what's right.

13. All fevers eventually come back to normal on the way to room tem perature.

14. There's always time sometime.

15. Common things are common.

16. He who turns to run away must first sign out AMA.

17. Uncommon manifestations of common diseases are more common than are uncommon diseases.

22. Death is a severe stage of shock, or shock is a pause in the act of dying.

23. It looks more like it does now than it did.

24. In medicine, always remember never to say always and never.

25. All bleeding is gross.

26. If you can't see it, it's probably not there.

27. Don't vomit on the doctor!

28. Remember, "Toast always falls jelly-side down."

29. If a patient has a catheter — he needs it.

30. Everyone gets treated exactly the same in here —-until he pisses you off.

31. The ER is a mixture of can do, can't do, and why the hell not!

32. To be right is only half the battle; to convince the patient is more dif ficult.

33. Remember, the problem is always better than the X-ray looks.

34. I was better, but I got over it.

35. WHY am I here?

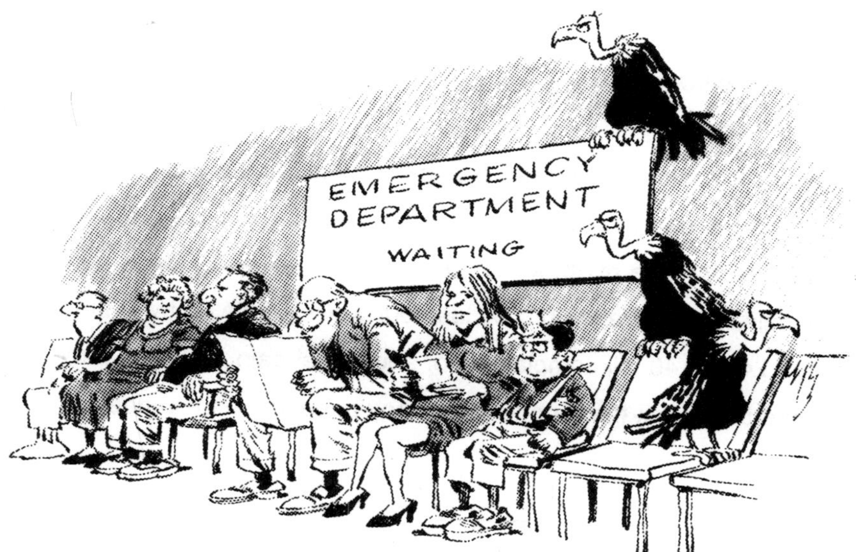

Math Quiz for ER Nurses

1. You are assisting a primary nurse with charcoal administration down an orogastric tube. The room measures eight feet by twelve feet. The patient starts to retch before the tube is pulled. Knowing that charcoal can spew out of a tube in a five foot radius (even with a thumb over the opening) and the stretcher is two feet wide, how many feet per second do you have to back up to get less charcoal on you than the primary nurse?

Write your answer here__________

2. Doctor A picks up a chart out of the rack. It is a repeat patient with abdominal pain. Doctor A puts the chart back. Doctor B picks up the chart five minutes later and also returns it to the rack. Doctor A leaves the nurses' station heading south at three miles per hour. Doctor B leaves the nurses station for the doctors' lounge at five miles per hour. How long before the patient is at equal distance from Doctor A and Doctor B?

Write your answer here__________

3. You were assigned two large treatment rooms and the GYN room. By the end of the day you have cared for ten patients. Four patients were female over the age of 80, all complaining of weakness. Two patients were male, ages 72 and 50. The last four were female, between the ages of 24 and 40, all complaining of abdominal pain. It is 3:00 p.m. and time to restock the rooms. How many bedpans will you need?

Write your answer here__________

4. You are the primary nurse for an elderly patient with congestive heart failure. The IV stick was exceptionally difficult, but you are able to start an 18 gauge catheter on the second attempt. You leave the room to check on another patient. A relative thinks that the IV has stopped dripping and opens the clamp. How much IV fluid will infuse before you return?

Write your answer here___________

5. You are sent for your morning coffee break. You need to use the restroom but can't find one unoccupied and have to walk down to the lobby. The coffee pot is dry and you have to make more. When you get to the cafeteria, the line extends ten feet into the hallway. You can't remember exactly when your break began. How much time do you have left?

Write your answer here___________

6. You are the primary nurse taking care of a particularly shy female in the gynecology room. Her private physician arrives to see her, but you can see that he is not in a particularly good mood. After much coaxing, the patient agrees to a pelvic exam. How many people will open the door during the exam?

Write your answer here___________

7. You have answered how many questions in this quiz so far? ___

You have been paged how many times since starting? ___

Total ___

Write your answer here___________

7. You are assigned to the EENT room. You have a patient to be checked for a peritonsillar abscess. The ENT physician has been paged and expects to arrive in 45 minutes. Three hours later, he arrives and is at the patient's side, asking for a flashlight. Lightly jogging at 22 miles per hour, how many rooms will you have to search before you find one?

Write your answer here__________

8. You have been asked to cover a coworker's rooms during her break. One of her patients is an elderly, confused male with an enlarged prostate. A catheter has been inserted and his physician is coming to see him. Somehow he manages to get off the stretcher. The drainage bag is firmly hooked to the side rail. Knowing that the catheter is 16 inches long and the drainage tubing is three feet long, will he be able to reach the door before pulling out the catheter?

Write your answer here__________

9. An elderly man arrives in the Emergency Department by rescue squad. Twenty minutes later his wife arrives and registers him. She is shown the entrance to the Department and slowly shuffles in. How many rooms will she walk into before she finds him?

Write your answer here__________

10. A college student named Muffy is brought to the Emergency Department with a sore throat. She has no relatives in the area. Will there be enough chairs in the waiting room for deeply concerned significant others? (+ or-) how many

Write your answer here__________

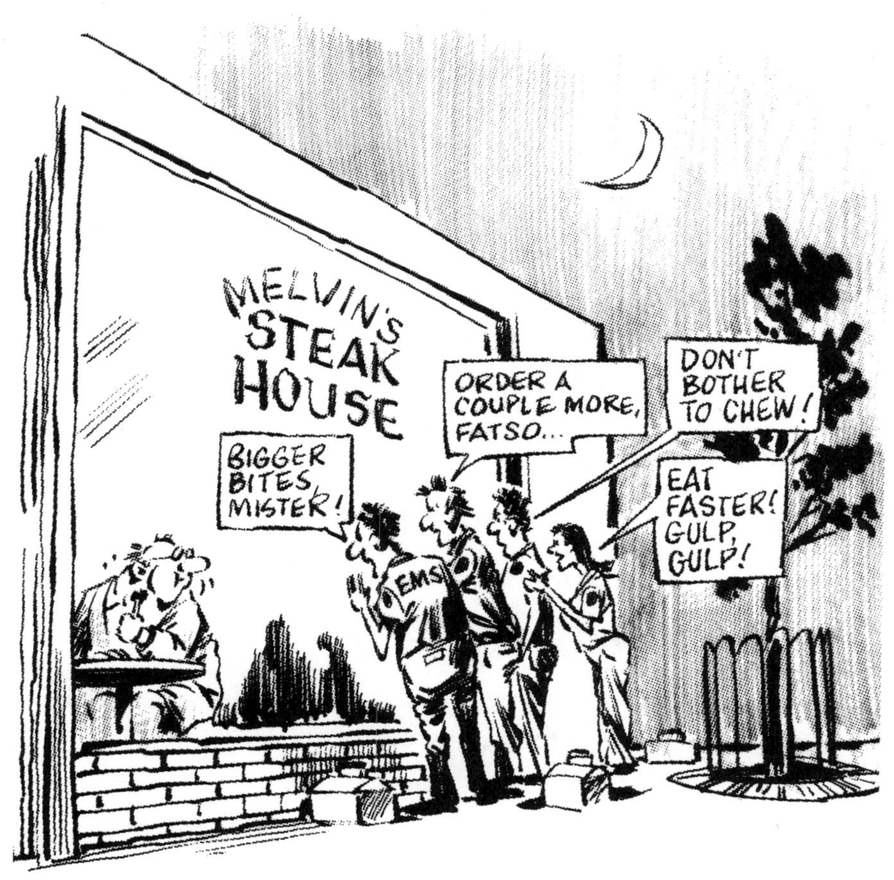

A pack of renegade EMT's on the prowl" Hal

You Might be an EMS Professional if...

- You are prone to complimenting complete strangers on their 'great veins' when you are out in public.
- Discussing dismemberment over a gourmet meal seems perfectly normal...
- Your idea of fine dining is anywhere you can sit down to eat...
- You get an almost irresistible urge to stand and wolf your food even in the nicest restaurants...
- You plan your dinner break while managing an overdose patient...
- Your diet consists of food that has gone through more processing than most computers...
- You believe chocolate is a food group...
- You refer to vegetables and are not talking about a food group...
- You believe a good tape job will fix anything...
- You have the bladder capacity of five people...
- Your idea of a good time is a full arrest at shift change...
- You believe in aerial spraying of Prozac...
- You firmly believe that if Dilantin, Haldol and Narcan were put in the water instead of floride, dentists may be busier but EMS would grind to a halt...
- You have your weekends off planned for a year in advance...
- Your idea of comforting a child includes placing them in a papoose restraint...
- You believe that "shallow gene pool" should be a recognized diagnosis...

- You believe that unspeakable evils will befall you if the phrase "Wow, it's really quiet" is uttered...

- You threaten to strangle anyone who even starts to say the "q" word when it is even remotely calm...

- You have ever referred to someone's death as a "Celestial Transfer"...

- You have ever referred to someone's death as a transfer to the "Eternal Care Unit"...

- You refer to someone in severe respiratory distress as a "smurf"...

- You feel that most suicide attempts should be given a free subscription to "Guns and Ammo" magazine...

- You have ever had a patient look you straight in the eye and say "I have no idea how that got stuck in there"...

- You have ever had to leave a patient's room before you begin to laugh uncontrollably...

- You think that caffeine should be available in I.V. form...

- You have ever restrained someone and it was not a sexual experience...

- You believe a "Supreme Being Consult" is your patients only hope...

- Your most common assessment question is "what changed tonight to make it an emergency after 6 (hours, days, weeks, months, years)?"...

- You have ever had a patient say, "but I'm not pregnant; I can't be pregnant; How can I be having a baby?"...

- Your bladder expands to the same size as a Winnebago's water tank...

- Your feet are slightly flatter and tougher than Fred Flintstone's...

- Your immune system is so well developed that it has been known to attack squirrels in the backyard...

- Your shoes have been seized and quarantined by the Centers for Disease Control in Atlanta...

- You believe that 90% of people are a poor excuse for proto plasm...

- You find humor in other people's stupidity...

- You disbelieve 90% of what you are told and 75% of what you see...

- You believe that the government should require a permit to repro duce...

- You believe that "too stupid to live" should be a diagnosis...

- Your favorite hallucinogenic is exhaustion...

- You believe your patient is demonically possessed...

- You have every referred to subcutaneous air as "Rice Krispies"...

- You have thought OD instead of BBQ when asked to get the Charcoal...

- You believe that a large part of your daily calorie requirement is provided by Tylenol, Advil, or Excedrin...

- You always try to schedule days off around phases of the moon...

- You believe that the sight of a full moon can ruin a perfectly good day...

- You find yourself avoiding an unhealthy looking "COPD"er in the grocery store in fear that he'll drop near you and you will have to do CPR on your day off ...

- Your family members have to have a fever of at least 105 or be missing a limb with active bleeding in order to receive your sympa thy...

- You've ever held a 14 gauge needle over someone's vein and said "now there's going to be a little poke"...

- You are the only one at the dinner table NOT allowed to talk about your day at work ...
- You've ever sworn that you were going to have "DNR" tatooed on your chest (or if you already have it tattooed)...
- You have ever considered MacDonalds as an appropriate and well balanced meal...
- You've ever had to restrain a parent (or significant other) so you could do your job...
- You have ever had to remind yourself that you can't cure stupidity...
- You automatically multiply by three the answer to the question "how many drinks did you have today?"...
- You get very, very scared when a child is "too" quiet...
- You are convinced that the amount of complaining by a patient is inversely proportional to how sick they are...
- You circle the dates of full moons in red on the calendar...
- You believe that there are some things that only a good autopsy can cure...
- You ever wanted to present the "poor-acting" award to a patient...
- You have ever included a nasopharyngeal airway as part of your evaluation of a patient's "unresponsiveness"...
- You calculate dopamine dosages in your head, but can't seem to balance your checkbook...
- Your social skills seem a little lacking, since most of your amusing anecdotes revolve around blood and vomit...
- You wonder what the big deal is when someone has a seizure...
- You refer to the Mega-code portion of ACLS as "the fun part"...
- You've ever said (to anyone) "so, did you find the fingers?"...

- You've ever had to contend with someone who thinks constipation for 4 hours is a medical emergency..
- You've ever entered a patient's chief complaint as "I'm drunk"...
- You refer to motorcyclists as "organ donors"...

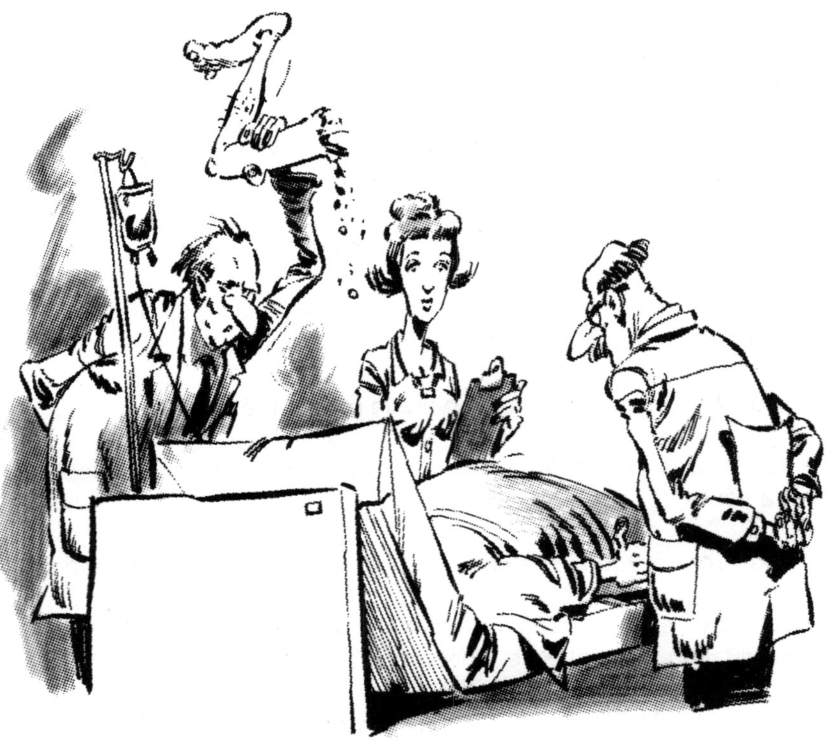

" Does it hurt when I do this?"

The "Veteran" EMT Reality Scale

(Note: A "yes" answer to any of the following statements makes it highly likely that you are a "veteran" EMT or Paramedic)
An abundance of "yes" answers makes it highly possible that you should be a contributor to the next edition of this book.

1. You now dispense meds based on the color of the label because you can't see the little letters anymore.
2. You feel like patting new probies on the head. 
3. Learning to do it wearing gloves is harder than learning to do it the first time.
4. You remember taking care of Quaalude OD's.
5. When you started, nobody had heard of "ACLS".
6. You are taking orders from doctors who used to be orderlies.
7. Your low back pain is worse than your patient who is on total disability and Medicare.
8. You can start IVs with your eyes closed... 'cuz you can't see those little veins anymore.
9. You don't work New Year's Eve anymore because you can't stay up that late.
10. You spend more time discussing your children's sex lives than your own.
11. You have oriented several new medics who have asked you how you've managed to survive for so long.
12. Dr. Scholl's products are a regular part of your shopping list.
13. "Man down" translates to you as: Drunk if unwitnessed, Seizure if witnessed.
14. "Been there-Done That" is your usual response, and it's the truth.

Top Ten Reasons Why We No Longer Call Them "Ambulance Drivers"

(found posted in local hospital)

10. The (hospital) EMS coordinator works very, very, very hard every day to keep a good working relationship between the EMS people and the hospital staff.

9. Modern day Paramedics actually know how to do more than drive an ambulance. They also know how to come in out of the rain. they know how to diagnose and treat lethal cardiac arrythmias. They know how to calculate and administer powerful IV medications using algebraic formulas while remembering every possible side effect, precaution, and adverse reaction. They know how to successfully perform an emergency surgical tracheostomy or needle chest decompression of a tension pneumothorax on a trauma patient at the side of the road in the dark during a thunderstorm.

8. Paramedics accept pay that is less than the average factory worker or gas meter reader to do the above day after day because they know that what they do in a days work will make a difference in someones life. Every day.

7. Paramedics do what nobody else is willing to do, such as carefully and respectfully picking up what is left of somebody's five year old child who died of a massive head injury caused by a drunk driver. And then take care of the drunk driver.

6. Paramedics now usually go to accredited college programs and go on to earn degrees from those institutions. They also find time on their days off to attend in-services, audits, review sessions, and courses such as ACLS, PALS, BTLS, etc. to constantly maintain their credentials as required by the National Registry .

5. Paramedics risk their lives daily by exposing themselves to blood and body fluids and have no way of knowing if those substances are contaminated with HIV, hepatitis, etc.

4. This hospitals EMS coordinator does not want, need, or deserve the harassment.

3. Paramedics can scoop up brain matter from the pavement or pick up a homeless alcoholic who has laid in his own excretement for three days, and then go to lunch and eat spaghetti with red sauce.

2. We want to believe that Paramedics are more than ambulance drivers - especially if they are called to restart our own hearts, rescue our own teenager from a submerged vehicle, or to delive our babies in an emergency.

1. They deserve our respect.

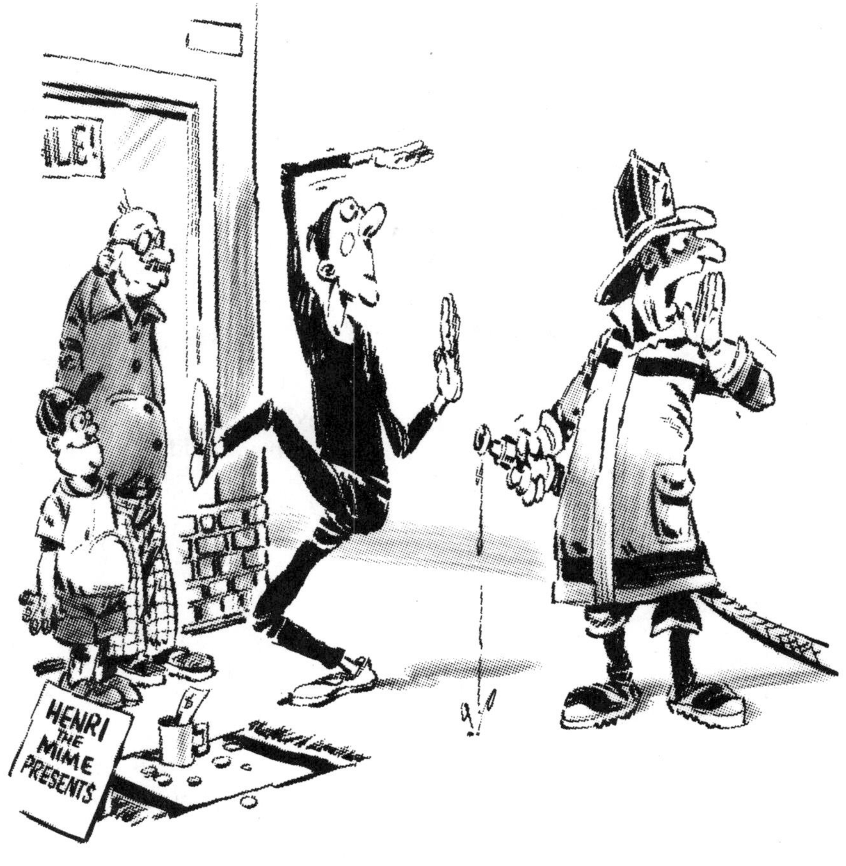

" Bring up the Jaws of Life...he's been trapped in there for over an hour'

Strange Complaints at the Scene

No matter what you have heard those in all aspects of Emergency Services can rest assured that you haven't "heard it all".

It is difficult for most of us to believe the stories we hear, but they sure do give us some laughs and we can't wait to share them with our counterparts.

We are sure that these complaints listed below will remind you of a few you have heard.

"My hands tingle when I take a dump"
(Are they sitting on their hands?)

Paramedic: "Do you have a heart condition?"
Patient: "Yes, I have a spacemaker"

"His fever got up to one-oh-three point twelve"

"I've been vomiting stuff that tastes like earwax"
(And how long have you been doing this comparitive study?)

"I haven't demonstrated in three months."

"I just got old timers disease"
(Alzheimer's disease)

"I don't think it's my heart, I don't have any pain, it just hurts."

A 20 y/o man complained of burning pain in his right thigh, and a foul odor. The EMT noted smoke coming from his pants leg. The patient reached in his pocket and pulled out a LIT cigarette and exclaimed "Damn, I thought I put that out!"

While examining an obese woman, a paramedic moved the patient's left breast to the side in order to listen to her heart. Beneath her breast he found a sandwich in a zip-lock bag. The patient stated "Oh yeah, I forgot about that."

"My vaginal discharge is so heavy that I have to change my underwear EVERYDAY!"

A thirteen year old girl complained of nausea and vomiting. She was found to be pregnant. She denied ever having had sex. When confronted with the fact that she had to have had sex to be pregnant (barring the possibility of a second emaculate conception) she said that she shares a bed with her older sister who often has sex with her boyfriend, and she "might have gotten splashed with some".

A 50 woman called 9-1-1 with complaints of a roach in her left ear. The woman had tried to wash it out of her left ear by pouring water in the right ear to "wash it through".

A 28 year old male was brought into the ER after an attempted suicide. He had swallowed several nitroglycerin tablest and a fifth of vodka. When asked about the bruises around his head and chest, he said they were from ramming himself into the wall in an attempt to make the nitroglycerin explode.

(Remember that we are compiling more of these unique complaints to share with you in Edition 2 of "Masters of Disasters". Send in your favorites and if we use it, we will send you a free copy of the 2nd Edition.)

It happened like this......
or
Accident Reporting 101

1. Coming home, I drove into the wrong house and collided with a tree I don't have.

2. The other car hit with me without giving me warning.

3. I thought my window was down, but it was up when I put my hand through it.

4. I hit a parked truck coming the other way.

5. A truck backed through my windshield into my wife's face.

6. That pedestrian hit me and went under my car.

7). That guy was all over the road, I had to swerve a few of times before I hit him.

8. I pulled away from the side of the road, looked at my mother-in-law and headed over the embankment.

9. When I tried to kill that fly, I drove into a telephone pole.

10. I was shopping for plants all day and on my way home, as I reached the intersection, a hedge sprang up, obscuring my vision.

11. I had been driving for 40 years when I fell asleep at the wheel and had an accident.

12. I was on my way to the doctors with rear end trouble, when my universal joints gave way, making me have the accident.

13. To avoid hitting the bumper of the car in front, I struck the pedestrian.

14. My car was legally parked as it backed into the other vehicle.

15. An [invisible] car came out of nowhere, struck my car and vanished.

16. I told the police that I was not injured, but when I removed my hat, I found I had a skull fracture.

17. I was sure the old man would not make it to the other side of the street when I struck him.

18. The telephone pole was approaching fast, I attempted to swerve out of it's way, when it struck the front of my car.

Working the long hours and often through the night,those in Emergency Services often rely on one of our most popular stimulants to keep them going. Just how much a role is played by the ever present cup of coffee was brought to light by the following poem, Posted on the bulletin board at the local hospital where the hospital, ambulance and police folks gather, we found the following:

A Caffeine Prayer

Caffeine is my shepherd, I shall not doze,
It maketh me to wake in green pastures.
It leadeth me beyond the sleeping masses,
It restoreth my buzz.

It leadeth me in the paths of consciousness for its name's sake.
Yea, though I walk through the valley of the shadow of addiction,
I will fear no Equal.

For thou art with me; thy cream and thy sugar they comfort me.
Thou preparest a carafe before me in the presence of Juan Valdez,
Thou anointest my day with pep; my mug runneth over.
Surely richness and taste shall follow me all the days of my life,

And I will dwell in the House of Folger's forever.

(PC Disclaimer)

The above was not a sneaky commericial effort on our part. as a matter of fact we urge you to use the coffee brand of your choice, as often as you please, wherever. alone or a with whomever you choose. No member of the staff or any of their family members are associated with any coffee grower, broker, distributor, retailer, advertising agency or anything else that could get us in trouble.

Checking Out

In the early days of EMS, a couple of paramedics were working a code with a real gung-ho Med Control Doc, on the other end of the radio. They had emptied the drug box into their patient, with no success. In desperation, they asked the Doc for further instructions. "Do you have a white pages phone book there?," asked the Doc. When they replied (puzzled) in the affirmative he told them "Then look him up and scratch his name out."

The charge nurse told the brand new intern that it required a physician to inform the family of an unsuccessful trauma code, that the patient had expired. The intern went to the crowded waiting area and asked if the Wilson family was present. He was immediately surrounded by a number of concerned relatives. When one lady identified herself as Mrs. Wilson, the new Dr. said, "Guess who died?"

When telemetry came into EMS we were given the explaination that having the magic box was like having the Dr. at your side. I wish the Dr. had been at the scene with the cardiac patient, his family and our crew one night.. Perhaps then he would have thought twice about interperting the rythm strip and blurting out for all to hear him say over the radio..."Stop working on him and start digging a hole"

The following has most recently been traveling the internet....like most of the information availible it may or may not be factual.....but there is no doubt that it is worth including....and hoping that it is true.....

The Littlest Firefighter

The 26-year old mother stared down at her son who was dying of terminal leukemia. Although her heart was filled with sadness, she also had a strong feeling of determination. Like any parent she wanted her son to grow up and fulfill all his dreams. Now that was no longer possible. The leukemia would see to that. But she still wanted her son's dreams to come true. She took her son's hand and asked, "Billy, did you ever think about what you wanted to be once you grew up? Did you ever dream and wish what you would do with your life? "Mommy, I always wanted to be a fireman when I grew up." Mom smiled back and said, "Let's see if we can make your wish come true,"

Later that day she went to her local fire department in Phoenix, Arizona, where she met Fireman Bob, Who had a heart as big as Phoenix. She explained her son's final wish and asked if it might be possible to give her six-year old son a ride around the block on a fire engine. Fireman Bob said, "Look, we can do better than that. If you'll have your son ready at seven o'clock Wednesday morning, we'll make him an honorary fireman for the whole day. He can come down to the fire station, eat with us, go out on all the calls, the whole nine yards! And if you'll give us his sizes, we'll get a real fire uniform for him, with a real fire hat -not a toy one- with the emblem of the Phoenix Fire Department on it, a yellow slicker like we wear and rubber boots. They're all manufactured right here in Phoenix, so we can get them fast."

Three days later Fireman Bob picked up Billy, dressed him in his fire uniform and escorted him from his hospital bed to the waiting hook and ladder truck. Billy got to sit on the back of the truck and help steer it back to the fire station. He was in heaven. There were three fire calls in Phoenix that day and Billy got to go out on all three calls. He rode in the different fire engines, the paramedic's van and even the fire chief's car. He was also video taped for the local news program.

Having his dream come true, with all the love and attention that was lavished upon him, so deeply touched Billy that he lived three months longer than any doctor thought possible. One night all of his vital signs began to drop dramatically and the head nurse, who believed in the hospice concept that no one should die alone, began to call the family members to the hospital.

Then she remembered the day Billy had spent as a fireman, so she called the fire chief and asked if it would be possible to send a fireman in uniform to the hospital to be with Billy as he made his transition. The chief replied, " We can do better than that. We'll be there in five minutes. Will you please do me a favor? When you hear the sirens screaming and see the lights flashing, will you announce over the PA system that there is not a fire?" It's just the fire department coming to see one of it's finest members one more time. And will you open the window to his room? Thanks."

About five minutes later a hook and ladder truck arrived at the hospital, extended it's ladder up to Billy's third floor open window and 16 firefighters climbed up the ladder into Bill's room. With his mother's permission, the hugged him and held him and told him how much they loved him. With his dying breath, Billy looked up at the fire chief and said, Chief, am I really a fireman now? "Billy, you are," the chief said. With those words, Billy smiled and closed his eyes one last time.

Just Another Day in EMS

I delivered a baby on the ambulance cot;
I baptized a newborn whose life ended before it began.

I hugged a frightened child;
I was kissed by an intoxicated old man.

I held the hand of a teenage girl as she delivered a 3-pound baby;
I listened to the mournful squeak of a stretcher being wheeled to the morgue.

I gently stroked the fragile hand of a 102 year old woman;
I hesitated at the outreached hand of a 300 pound prisoner in handcuffs.

I turdged for 10 hours in my boots;
I had a teenager vomit on those same boots.

I rubbed the feverish body of a 14 year old cancer patient;
I cradled the ice-cold hand of a child hit by a car.

I was referred to as "an angel of mercy";
I was called every four-letter word in the book.

I always see fear in people's eyes;
I almost never see joy or relief.

I listened to a tormented voice pleading for the preservation of life;
I heard the threatening words of one bent on self-destruction.

I spoke with the girl who was hoping she had the flu, not a pregnancy;
I see innocent people hurt or killed by a drunk driver, and the drunk driver is never hurt.

I marveled at the genius of a cardiologist;
I saw a 12 year old boy who shot himself in the head, and the gun was still loaded at his feet.

I talked in circles with a schizophrenic person;
I was horrified at the battered body of a child whose parents were incapable of love.

I gazed at a horribly burned body;
I shuddered at a cold water drowning.

I see women beaten up by their spouses, but they never press charges;
I walk into houses and do CPR with family watching over my shoulder in tears.

I arrive at serious auto accidents, and the first words I hear are, "Am I going to die?";
I find out hours later they did die.

I listen to the repeated question, "Why?", from a family devestated by death;
I search my soul for the answers to their question.

This is just another day in EMS.

When God made Paramedics.........

When the Lord made Paramedics, he was into his sixth day of overtime when an angel appeared and said, "You're doing a lot of fiddling around on this one." And The Lord said, "Have you read the Specs on this order?

A paramedics has to be able to carry an injured person up a wet grassy hill in the dark, dodge stray bullets to reach a dying child unarmed, enter homes with barley enough room to move, and console a grieving mother as he is doing CPR on a baby he knows will never breath again."

"He has to be in top mental condition at all times, running on no sleep, black coffee and half-eaten meals. And he has to have six pairs of hands.

The angel shook her head slowly and said, "Six pairs of hands...no way."

"It's not the hands that are causing me problems," said the Lord, "It's the three pairs of eyes the medic has to have."

"That's on the standard model? Asked the angel.

The Lord nodded. "One pair that sees open sores as he's drawing blood and asks the patient if they may be HIV positive." (When he already knows and wishes he'd taken that accounting job.)
"Another pair here in the side of his head for his partners safety. And another pair of eyes here in front that can look reassuringly at a bleeding victim and say, You'll be alright ma'am when he knows it isn't so."

"Lord," said the angel, touching his sleeve, "rest and work on this tomorrow."

"I can't said the Lord, "I already have a model that can talk a 250 pound drunk out from behind a steering wheel without incident and feed a family of five on a private service check."

The angel circled the model of the paramedic very slowly, "Can it think? she asked.

"You bet," said the Lord. "It can tell you the symptoms of 100 illnesses; recite drug calculations in it's sleep: intubate, defibrillate, medicate and continue CPR nonstop over terrain that any doctor would fear. and still it keeps it's sense of humor.

This medic also has phenomenal personal control. He can deal with a multi-victim trauma, coax a frightened elderly person to unlock their door, comfort a murder victim's family, and then read in the daily paper how paramedics were unable to locate a house quickly enough, allowing the person to die. A house which had no street sign, no house numbers, no phone to call back."

Finally, the angel bent over and ran her finger across the cheek of the paramedic. "There's a leak," she pronounced. "I told you that you were trying to put to much into this model."

"That's not a leak," said the Lord, "It's a tear."

"What's the tear for? Asked the angel.

It's for bottled-up emotions, for patients they've tried in vain to save, for commitment to that hope that they will make a difference in a person's chance to survive, for life."

"You're a genius," said the angel.

The Lord looked somber. "I didn't put it there," He said.

A Letter to The Insurance Company

Superior Health Insurance
ATTN: Claims Review
1234 W. Main St.
New York, NY 90610

Dear Sirs:

This letter is in response to your recent letter requesting a more detailed explanation concerning my recent ER visit at Medical Hospital. Specifically, you asked for an expansion in reference to Block 21(a)(3) of the claim form (reason for hospital visit). On the original form, I put "Stupidity". I realize now that this answer was somewhat vague and so I will attempt to more fully explain the circumstances leading up to my hospitalization.

I had just finished a quick bite to eat at the local burger joint and needed to use the restroom. I entered the bathroom, took care of my business, and just prior to the moment in which I had planned to raise my trousers, the locked case that prevents theft of the toilet paper in such places came undone and, feeling it striking my knee, unthinkingly, I immediately, and with unnecessary force, returned the lid back to its normal position.

Unfortunately, as I did this I also turned, and certain parts of my body, which were still exposed, were trapped between the device's lid and its main body. Feeling such intense and immediate pain caused me to jump back. It quickly came to my attention that, when one's privates are firmly attached to an unmovable object, it is not a good idea to jump in the opposite direction.

Upon recovering some of my senses, I attempted to reopen the lid. However, my slamming of it had been sufficient to allow the locking mechanism to engage. I then proceeded to get a hold on my pants and subsequently removed my keys from them. I intended to try to force the lock of the device open with one of my keys; thus extracting myself.

Unfortunately, when I attempted this, my key broke in the lock. Embarrassment of someone seeing me in this unique position became a minor concern, and I began to call for help in as much of a calm and rational manner as I could. An employee from the restaurant quickly arrived and decided that this was a problem requiring the attention of the store manager.

Betty, the manager, came quickly. She attempted to unlock the device with her keys. Since I had broken my key off in the device, she could not get her key in. Seeing no other solution, she called the EMS (as indicated on your form in block 21(b)(1)).

After approximately 15 minutes, the EMS arrived, along with two police officers, a fire-rescue squad, and the channel 4 ``On-the-Spot'' news team. The guys from the fire department quickly took charge as this was obviously a rescue operation.

The senior member of the team discovered that the device was attached with bolts to the cement wall that could only be reached once the device was unlocked. His discovery was by means of tearing apart the device located in the stall next to the one that I was in. (Since the value of the property destroyed in his examination was less than $50 (my deductible) I did not include it in my claim.) His partner, who seemed like an intelligent fellow at the time, came up with the idea of cutting the device from the wall with the propane torch that was in the rescue truck.

The fireman went to his truck, retrieved the torch, and commenced to attempt to cut the device from the wall. Had I been in a state to think of such things, I might have realized that in cutting the device from the wall several things would also inevitably happen. First, the air inside of the device would quickly heat up, causing items inside the device to suffer the same effects that are normally achieved by placing things in an oven. Second, the metal in the device is a good conductor of heat causing items that are in contact with the device to react as if thrown into a hot skillet. And, third, molten metal would shower the inside of the device as the torch cut through.

The one bright note of the propane torch was that it did manage to cut, in the brief time that I allowed them to use it, a hole big enough for a small pry bar to be placed inside of the device. The EMS team then loaded me, along with the device, into the waiting ambulance as stated on your form.

Due the small area of your block 21(a)(3), I was unable to give a full explanation of these events, and thus used the word which I thought best described my actions that led to my hospitalization.

Sincerely,
Mr. Smith

On the Way Home

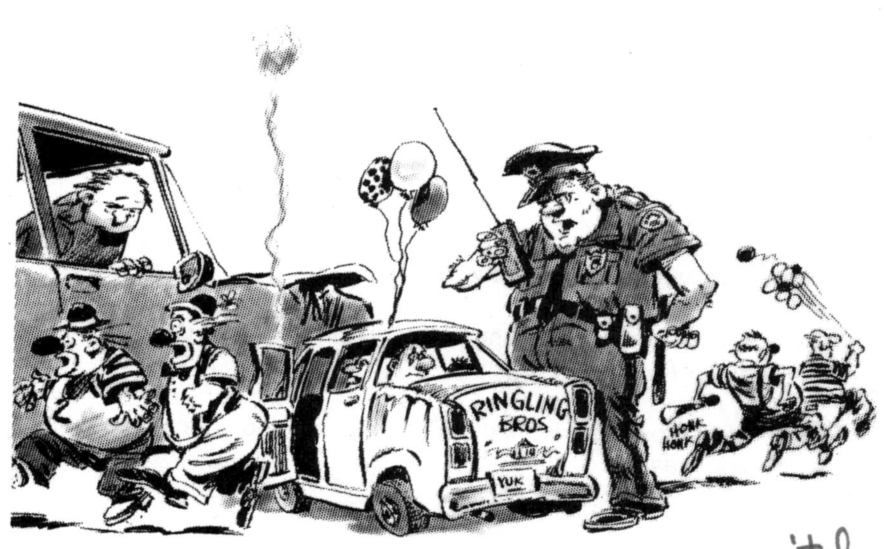

" You can cancel the ambulance, it doesn't look like anything serious"

You Know You've Been in EMS Too Long When ...

1. Your version of a slinky negligee is a sweatsuit with short sleeves.

2. The word "Code" is now an unwelcome four-letter word in your vocabulary.

3. When family emergencies are classified as: Code 1 - Not urgent but needs attention; Code 2 - Urgent and needs your attention ASAP; Code 3 - Urgent and needs your attention NOW!.

4. When SOB now means Shortness Of Breath, and not necessarily how you feel about a person.

5. When you stop looking at clothing for fashion, and look at it for function and durability.

6. When your spouse has his or her hands on you, and the reason is practicing Patient Assessment, and not passion.

7. When you're on duty, and your only child doesn't recognize your voice on the phone.

8. When you're on duty, and go home, your own dog won't let you into the family house, because it no longer recognizes you.

9. When members of the opposite sex are on the same vehicle in vari ous states of half-dress, and nobody notices enough to mention it, or be embarrassed.

10. When the word "tone" doesn't refer to color, but that sound that sends your entire body into overdrive.

11. When the colors red, white and blue bring to mind accident scenes, and then the American Flag.

12. When "latex" no longer immediately brings to mind safe sex, but the gloves you wear.

13. When it takes you longer to set up your gear and get into the show er, than it does to actually take the shower.

14. When you take time off, you're more nervous than when you're "on duty."

15. When every time you're a passenger in a POV, you call out, "Clear to the right!" at every intersection.

16. When "PEARL" isn't something you wear around your neck, but is something you pray you'll see in your patient's eyes.

17. When it becomes normal to drop your fork and run out on family meals, get-togethers, and company ... and those left in your wake understand and continue, as this is perfectly normal behavior among civilized people.

18. When family pets clear a path when they hear the tones go off, so they won't get mowed over, then greet you when you come home, forgiving you for doing just that.

19. When you are asleep, and dream the tones are going off, and you wake up heading for the bedroom door in a full run, shoes on, radio in hand, and you don't even recall getting out of bed.

20. When "TIME" means how long it took you to reach your patient's home instead of what hour of the day it is.

21. When "RHYTHM" is a designation of heart function, and no longer a birth control method.

22. When matters of the heart refer to CPR, not romance.

23. When "VENTILATE" means breathing for your patient, and not opening doors and windows.

24. When caffeine becomes a SEDATIVE.

25. When you shake a person's hand, and your first thought is "Great veins!"

26. When joules (pronounced "jewels") are not diamonds and emeralds, but the power rate on a Defibrillator unit.

27. When "Circling the Drain" has nothing to do with water emptying from your bathtub or sink.

28. When sticks aren't what fall from trees and litter your lawn, but what you do to a patient's veins.

29. When hairline refers to a fracture, and not a concern for your barber.

30. When reflective tape becomes a fashion plus.

31. When artifact is something you see on a Defibrillator unit, and not an antique you find in a museum.

32. When a motionless and silent child is no longer a desired sight.

33. When a male purchases sanitary napkins, not for his wife, but for pressure dressings on his patients.

34. When MAST refers to anti-shock pants, and not something that attaches the sails to your boat...which you no longer have time for anyway.

35. When a "FIB" was bad to tell your mom, and now it's a bad rhythm f or your patient.

36. When you no longer watch sporting events to see the scores, but to see how the EMS people on-scene handle the trauma cases.

37. When you realize just what is meant by "There is no sex in EMS"...and so does your significant other.

38. When "P.O." no longer necessarily means you are angry at some thing.

39. When A&P isn't a grocery store's name anymore, but is Anatomy and Physiology to you.

40. When "RADIAL" is where your patient's pulse is located, not what type tires are on your vehicle.

41. When the "best funny line" expression about how cold your hands are finally results in one of your patients asking you, "And just how did you find out how cold a bullfrog's butt is???"

42. When the majority of your patients are no longer your parent's age, but are your own children's age.

43. When you notice that your worst "Pre-EMS bad hair day" isn't even close to your very best "EMS hair day"...and neither you nor your partner mentions it or are embarrassed by it anymore.

44. When you are traveling down the road in your car and reach a per son on the cell phone and the first words out of your mouth tend to be, "We are presently enroute to your facility with..."

45. You can finish a seven-course dinner before anyone else has touched their salad.

46. You sleep fully dressed at home, just because you like to.

47. The phone at home rings, and you put your shoes on.

48. You have a pet name for your cardiac monitor.

49. Your idea of a great dinner is one that's warm.

50. Your spouse takes you to dinner at a nice restaurant and you tell the maitre'd that you'd like it fixed to go "just in case."

51. You can type Med Control's phone number faster than your own ... without looking.

52. You know the patient's medical history better than they do.

53. You drive better asleep than you do awake.

54. You can eat spaghetti and meatballs while watching "The Texas Chainsaw Massacre."

55. You wake up for a shift change and can't remember the calls you ran last night.

56. You talk to your ambulance.

57. You no longer get upset when someone calls you an "Ambulance Driver."

58. Your idea of a good call is one that's cancelled while you're enroute.

59. When starting your personal vehicle, you reach for the "Battery On" switch.

60. You buy stock in Wendy's and McDonald's just to try and get the "shareholder's discount."

61. Your Christmas wish list only includes items from Gall's, Dyna-Med and Laerdal catalogues.

62. You refer to "Third Watch" as "educational television."

63. Your spouse sleeps with their mouth open, and you see it as a great chance to practice your intubation technique.

T-Shirts Seen Leaving the Station

Tee shirts have become a National and International way of representing ourselves and expressing a message to those we encounter. Unfortunately it is not a message that we can turn on and off.
Many of those listed below may give a positive or negative image, but they are out there...'cause we have seen them .

"Coed Naked EMS: Only the Tough can do a code in the buff"

"Coed Naked Firefighting : FInd Em Hot and Leave 'Em Wet"

"Coed Naked Nursing: Your butt is ours"
(with the crossed needles in front of the Star of Life)

"Coed Naked EMS: It takes big balls to run a code in the buff!!"

"Volunteers do it for free!"

"Search & Rescue Officers do it any time, any place, under any conditions and they do it for free."

"They pay us sh*t, but where else can you have so much fun?"

"Bad planning on your part does not constitute an emergency on my part"

"Support your local Search and Rescue Squad - Get Lost".

"Practice safer sex - sleep with a paramedic"

"Sleep safe - put a fire detector on your door and a paramedic in your bed"

"Support your local medical examiner - Die Strangely"

"Paramedics Save Lives - EMT Skills Save Paramedics"

"Paramedics Save Lives - EMTs Carry the Jump Kits"

"Sometimes you need a good paddling" (picture of EMT-P defibig ing a body on the floor)

A tree with a cat on top and a firefighter climbing a ladder to rescue the cat: “Firemen would do anything for a pussy”.

“Firefighters have longer hoses!”

“Firefighters pull their own hose.”

“P A R A M E D I C
On the street or in the bedroom, it’s called the GOLDEN HOUR for a reason!!!”

“Brains and blood, Guts and sh*t. We’ll be there, When you get hit!”

Paramedics have longer on-scene times.

“911 makes [Paramedics/EMTs] come.”

“Sometimes a good paddling is all you need to get you back in l line!” (Shown with picture of EKG of VFib converting to Normal Sinus Rhythm, and defib paddles below)

“Dial 911- because shit happens!”

“Step Into My Office” (showing a fully involved fire)

“Thanks to [insert favorite EMS level here] the beat goes on.”

“My paramedic gives me a charge”

“Shock ‘em, make ‘em jump, get a rhythm, and a pump!”

“Less than 8, intubate!” (GCS)

“O2 is good, blue is bad!”

“Just another slave to the great God “Motorola”

“You’re just jealous cuz the voices talk to <u>me</u>.” (On a Fire Dispatcher’s shirt)

Please Accept That

To The One I Love,

I became involved in emergency service work because there is a need for people to help others who are in trouble. Sometimes there are calls I respond to , however, that are difficult to talk about - even with the person you love and trust the most in the world.

Please accept that.

There are at times experiences I suffer which hurt me very deeply, and I might bring my suffering home. Sometimes my feelings bother me so much so that I can't even talk about them. Maybe it's because I don't want you to even imagine what I've suffered, or maybe it's because I'm afraid that you won't fully understand the depth of my feelings. During these times I'll become moody or irritable, and I may not seem to care much about your feelings or problems.

Please accept that.

You love me for who and what I am. I choose to do what I do because it's so important to me and to those I help, and although it's sometimes very difficult and maybe even dangerous, I love doing what I do, and I do it well. In short, I'm proud of what I am, and I hope that you are proud of me.

There are scenes, though, when I feel that I didn't do enough - so many people out there depend upon me; there are even times I get frustrated and even angry at my co-workers, myself, even the victims of tragedy. There are times that the horrors I have to deal with just overwhelm me. That's when I have to sort things out by myself or with others who were there with me.

Please accept that.

So, please, if I have a really bad call and just can't talk, it isn't because I don't love and care for you. It's not because I doubt your love and concern for me. I'm just not ready to open up. When this happens, don't try to understand - just accept the fact that I'm hurting and that I'll talk to you when I can.

I promise.

The Christmas Holiday's

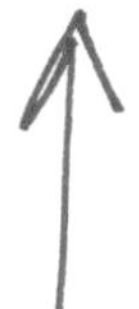

An EMS Christmas

'Twas the night before Christmas & all through our town,
Ambulances sat quietly - call volume was down.
The firehouse manning, without any calls,
All settled cozily within station walls.

The city grew silent as the night grew so deep;
My partner and I settled in for some sleep.
But no sooner dreaming in our beds were we,
When ECC woke us, crying, "Hurry! Car against tree!"

The call had come in for a bad MVA;
Some nutcase claimed he'd hit Santa's sleigh!
"Head trauma," we thought, as we gathered our gear,
"Or maybe a drunk driver - it's that time of year."

As we raced to the scene with our sirens and lights,
We hoped for the best, tonight of all nights.
We had no idea we were in for a surprise
And, on our arrival, couldn't believe our own eyes.

I said to my partner, "This must be a trick!
That man in the ditch just can't be St. Nick!"
A smashed-up sleigh! Toys thrown far and near!
And off to the side, a group of reindeer!

The driver of the car, with a bump on his head
Was crying and told us he wished he was dead.
"Oh, why did I have that one extra beer?
Now I've killed Santa - no Christmas <u>this</u> year!"

By now we'd decided that this was too strange,
So we tried to get backup, but were way out of range.
"No radio contact," to my partner I said,
"I'll check that one while you dress this one's head."

I approached the man in the ditch with great care.
He was dressed so oddly - he gave me a scare.
He wore a red suit and a strange kind of hat.
I thought to myself, "Who dresses like that?"

Then he opened his eyes and said, "Do not fear.
Just please help me up - I must catch my reindeer."
I said, "The reindeer are fine, but stay where you are.
You've taken a pretty hard hit from that car."

I didn't want to leave him, so I let out a holler:
"We're gonna need backboard, blanket roll and collar!"
As we worked, the man cried, "No! Please don't strap me down.
I have toys to deliver all over the town!
All of the children are depending on me
To get their presents under the Christmas tree."

"I'm sorry," I told him, as I shook my head sadly,
"You're going to the hospital - you've been hurt too badly."
He looked up at me and wiped away a tear
And told me, "Then you must bring the Christmas presents this year!"

"Visit every child's home in this town?" asked I.
"Sir, you must think I can make an ambulance fly!"
I thought I had made a serious blunder,
For his eyes grew steely, and his voice was like thunder.

"Now Dasher, now Dancer, now Prancer and Vixen,
Come Comet and Cupid and Donner and Blitzen!
Hitch onto that truck and take to the sky
For tonight, indeed, an ambulance will fly!"

I just shook my head as we loaded him in,
Then climbed in the cab, I just had to grin.
There were the reindeer, all in a row,
In front of the truck - we were ready to go.

"That's very cute," I thought. "I'll just go around."
But then they took off and our wheels left the ground!
Away we went, up over the trees,
Sailing along as light as a breeze.

We touched down on rooftops, delivering toys,
Dropping off gifts for good girls and boys.
We stopped in the hospital's ambulance bay
And wheeled him to the ER - and hoped that he'd stay.

"We'll call in later," we said on our way.
"This man's turned our ambulance into a sleigh!"
Then off we flew, all through the night,
Delivering toys til the dawn's first light.

Finally, at our station, we headed down,
Both of us happy to be on the ground.
The Chief was so mad, but the more we explained,
The less they believed us and the more they looked pained.
So we sat in our quarters - boy, were we in trouble!
We turned on the news and perked up on the double.

As the TV crews interviewed people in town,
It seems that some very strange things had gone down.
Tire tracks were found on a rooftop or two
And children said, "This year, Santa wore blue!"

I grinned at my partner and said, "It's no mystery!
This Christmas will go down in EMS history!"

The 12 Calls of Christmas

by Capt. Lisa K. Larson, RN, NREMTP

On the first call of Christmas, the Dispatcher sent to me:
One perky, brand-new EMT

On the second call of Christmas, the Dispatcher sent to me:
Two cut fingers, and one perky, brand-new EMT

On the third call of Christmas, the Dispatcher sent to me:
Three fender benders, two cut fingers, and one perky, brand-new EMT

On the fourth call of Christmas, the Dispatcher sent to me:
Four "One down's," three fender benders, two cut fingers, and one not-so-perky, not-so-new EMT

On the fifth call of Christmas, the Dispatcher sent to me:
Five pregnant women, four "One down's," three fender benders, two cut fingers, and one distressed, "when-does-it-stop?" EMT

On the sixth call of Christmas, the Dispatcher sent to me:
Six broken hips, five pregnant women, four "One down's," three fender benders, two cut fingers, and one scared, "What am I doing here?" new EMT

On the seventh call of Christmas, the Dispatcher sent to me:
Seven hypothermias, six broken hips, five pregnant women, four "One down's,"
three fender benders, two cut fingers, and one scared, "What am I doing here?" new EMT

On the eighth call of Christmas, the Dispatcher sent to me:
Eight working codes, seven hypothermias, six broken hips, five pregnant women, four "One down's," three fender benders, two cut fingers, and one ready-to-bail, getting older EMT

On the ninth call of Christmas, the Dispatcher sent to me:
Nine upset stomachs, eight working codes, seven hypothermias, six broken hips, five pregnant women, four "One down's," three fender benders, two cut fingers,
And one ready-to-bail, getting older EMT

On the tenth call of Christmas, the Dispatcher sent to me:
Ten frostbitten fingers, nine upset stomachs, eight working codes, seven hypothermias, six broken hips, five pregnant women, four "One down's," three fender benders, two cut fingers, and one overwhelmed, ready-to-leave EMT

On the eleventh call of Christmas, the Dispatcher sent to me:
Eleven hours of overtime, ten frostbitten fingers, nine upset stomachs, eight working codes, seven hypothermias, six broken hips, five pregnant women, four "One down's," three fender benders, two cut fingers, and one overwhelmed, "I'm-outta-here" EMT

On the twelfth call of Christmas, the Dispatcher sent to me:
Twelve minutes to eat, eleven hours of overtime, ten frostbitten fingers, nine upset stomachs, eight working codes, seven hypothermias, six broken hips, five pregnant women, four "One down's," three fender benders, two cut fingers, and one perky, brand-new EMT

Christmas Tunes for the Psychiatrically Challenged

SCHIZOPHRENIA: Do you hear what I hear?

MULTIPLE PERSONALITY DISORDER: We Three Queens Disoriented Are

DEMENTIA: I Think I'll be Home for Christmas

NARCISSISTIC: Hark the Herald Angels Sing About Me

MANIC: Deck the Halls and Walls and House and Lawn and Streets and Stores and Offices and Towns and Cars and Trucks, and Trees........

PARANOID: Santa Claus is Coming to Get Me

PERSONALITY DISORDER: You Better Watch Out, I'm Gonna Cry, I'm Gonna Pout, Maybe I'll Tell You Why

DEPRESSION: Silent Anedonia, Holy Anedonia, All is Flat, All is Lonely

OBSESSIVE-COMPULSIVE DISORDER: Jingle Bell, Jingle Bell, Jingle Bell Rock, Jingle Bell, Jingle Bell, Jingle Bell Rock, Jingle Bell, Jingle Bell, Jingle Bell Rock, Jingle Bell, Jingle Bell, Jingle Bell Rock, Jingle Bell, Jingle Bell, Jingle Bell Rock, Jingle Bell, Jingle Bell, Jingle Bell Rock, Jingle Bell, Jingle Bell, Jingle Bell Rock, Jingle Bell, Jingle Bell, Jingle Bell Rock, Jingle Bell, Jingle Bell, Jingle Bell Rock, Jingle Bell, Jingle Bell, Jingle Bell Rock Jingle Bell, Jingle Bell, Jingle Bell Rock, Jingle Bell, Jingle Bell, Jingle Bell Rock, Jingle Bell, Jingle Bell, Jingle Bell Rock, Jingle Bell, Jingle Bell, Jingle Bell Rock, Jingle Bell, Jingle Bell, Jingle Bell Rock, Jingle Bell, Jingle Bell, Jingle Bell Rock, Jingle Bell, Jingle Bell, Jingle Bell Rock,Jingle Bell, Jingle Bell, Jingle Bell Rock, Jingle Bell, Jingle Bell, Jingle Bell Rock, Jingle Bell, Jingle Bell, Jingle Bell Rock, Jingle Bell, Jingle Bell, Jingle Bell Rock, Jingle Bell, Jingle Bell, Jingle Bell Rock, Jingle Bell, Jingle Bell, Jingle Bell Rock, Jingle Bell, Jingle Bell, Jingle Bell Rock,Jingle Bell, Jingle Bell, Jingle Bell Rock, Jingle Bell, Jingle Bell, Jingle Bell Rock, Jingle Bell, Jingle Bell, Jingle Bell Rock, Jingle Bell, Jingle Bell, Jingle Bell Rock, Jingle Bell, Jingle Bell, Jingle Bell Rock, Jingle Bell, Jingle Bell, Jingle Bell Rock, Jingle Bell, Jingle Bell, Jingle Bell Rock,Jingle Bell, Jingle Bell, Jingle Bell Rock, Jingle Bell, Jingle Bell, Jingle Bell Rock, Jingle Bell, Jingle Bell, Jingle Bell Rock, Jingle Bell, Jingle Bell, Jingle Bell Rock, Jingle Bell, Jingle Bell, Jingle Bell Rock, Jingle Bell, Jingle Bell, Jingle Bell Rock, Jingle Bell, Jingle Bell, Jingle Bell Rock,Jingle Bell, Jingle Bell, Jingle Bell Rock, Jingle Bell, Jingle Bell, Jingle Bell Rock, Jingle Bell, Jingle Bell, Jingle Bell Rock, Jingle Bell, Jingle Bell, Jingle Bell Rock, Jingle Bell, Jingle Bell, Jingle Bell Rock, Jingle Bell, Jingle Bell, Jingle Bell Rock,Jingle Bell, Jingle Bell, Jingle Bell Rock, Jingle Bell, Jingle Bell, Jingle Bell Rock, Jingle Bell, Jingle Bell, Jingle Bell Rock, Jingle Bell, Jingle Bell, Jingle Bell Rock, Jingle Bell, Jingle Bell, Jingle Bell Rock, Jingle Bell, Jingle Bell, Jingle Bell Rock, Jingle Bell, Jingle Bell, Jingle Bell Rock,Jingle Bell, Jingle Bell, Jingle Bell Rock, Jingle Bell, Jingle Bell, Jingle Bell Rock, Jingle Bell, Jingle Bell, Jingle Bell Rock, Jingle Bell, Jingle Bell, Jingle Bell Rock, Jingle Bell, Jingle Bell, Jingle Bell Rock, (start over at the beginning......)

PASSIVE-AGGRESSIVE PERSONALITY: On The First Day of Christmas, My True Love Sent to Me ... (and Then He Took it all Back)

BORDERLINE PERSONALITY DISORDER: Thoughts of Roasting on an Open Fire

ALZHEIMERS
"What child is this?"

The Burned Out Christmas

T'was the night before Christmas and all through the station,
everyone's bitching who's not on vacation.
There is no stocking hung and nobody cares,
you may find some candy in the cushions of the chairs.

The morale is as high as a centipedes chin,
waiting in limbo for the crap to begin.
And right on schedule the alarm starts to sing,
we need to go pick up a drunk ding-a-ling.

After running all night we then get to bed,
puff up our pillows and descend our heads.
My partner lets out one hell of a yawn,
you'd be stupid to wake him until it is dawn.

And suddenly there's a knock at the door,
it's Santa Claus and its quarter to four.
"I demand that you patch up my thumb right away",
"so I can get on with the rest of my day".

So, needless to say I had to be rude,
to this pot-bellied ass with the attitude.
No one wakes us in the middle of the night,
and is rude and demanding and don't get a fight.

We dragged him inside by his curly short hairs,
and beat him senseless on the lazy boy chair.
We then got a call in the middle of the bout,
"by sleigh and raindeer the Ambulance is in route".

Assorted (Sick) Humor

A woman complains of bad knee pains to the paramedic. The medic questions her, "There must be something you're doing that you haven't told me. Can you think of anything that might be doing this to your knees?" "Well," she said a little sheepishly, "my husband and I have sex doggy-style on the floor every night." "That's got to be it," said the medic. "There are plenty of other positions and ways to have sex, you know." "Not if you're going to watch T.V. there ain't," she replied.

Paramedic (calling the ER): "How is that little boy doing, the one we brought in who swallowed ten quarters?" Nurse: "No change yet."

A Paramedic arrived at a semi concious Patient who had O/D on drugs, There was also a Police Officer at the scene who promptly asked the P/M why he had his finger up the patients Rectum to which came the reply "I am going to make him Vomit ".The Police Officer looked very puzzled and said "Sticking your finger up his rectum wont make him vomit will it?"the Paramedic replied "No, But you watch what happens when I stick it down his Throat".

I responded to a possible deceased the other day..On scene it was painfully obvious the elderly lady had been dead for QUITE some time. I inquired to the husband..who was obviously oblivious as to the chronic state of his wife.."What finally made you realize something as wrong?" To which he replied "The sex was the same but the damn dishes kept piling up!"

Q: What do you do with a seizure patient who's found in the bathtub?
A: Throw in your laundry.

A fireman looked out of the fire house window and noticed a little boy playing on the sidewalk. He had his red wagon, and he had hung small ladders on the side of it, and coiled the garden hose up in it, and he was wearing a fireman's hat. He had the wagon tied to his dog, so that the dog could pull the wagon. The fireman thought this was really cute, so he went out and told the little boy what a great looking fire truck he had. As he did, he noticed that the dog was tied to the wagon by his testicles. The fireman said, "Son, I don't want to try to tell you how to run your fire company or anything, but I think if you would tie that rope around your dog's neck you would go faster. "Maybe so, " said the boy, "But then I'd lose my siren!"

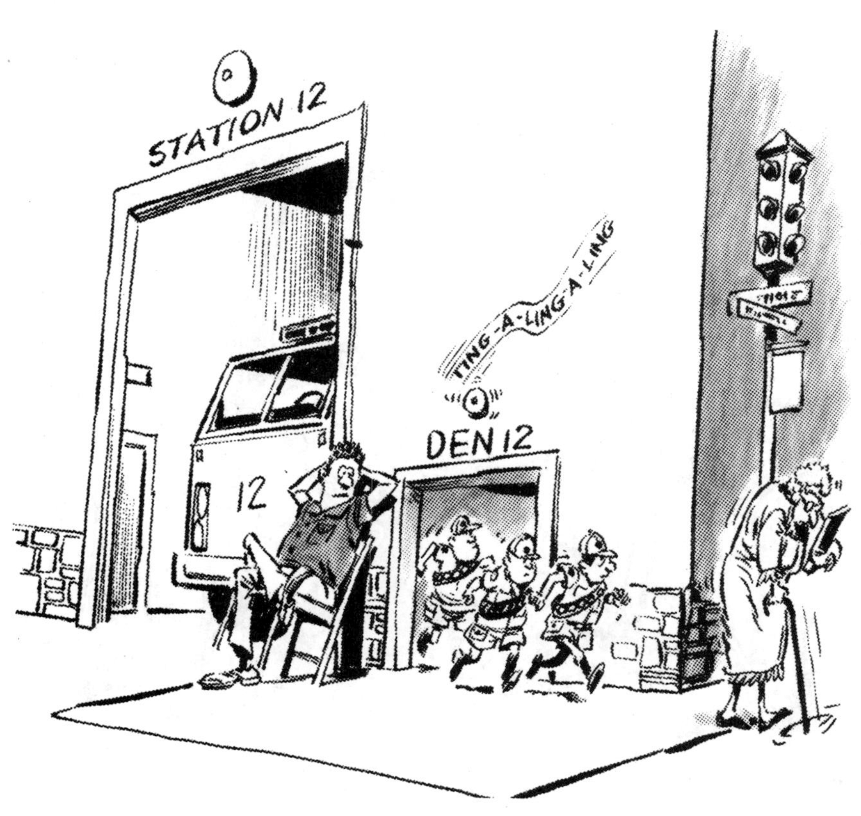

"Junior Firefighters"

A man swallowed a mouse while sleeping on the couch one day. His wife quickly called 9*1*1 and said, “Please come quickly. My husband just swallowed a mouse and he’s gagging and thrashing about.” “They’ll be right over,” the 911 dispatcher said. “In the meantime, keep waving a piece of cheese over his mouth to try to attract the mouse up and out of there.” When the paramedics arrived, they saw the wife waving a piece of smoked herring over her husband’s mouth. “Uhh, didn’t they tell you to use cheese, not herring, to lure the mouse.” “I know,” she replied, “but first I’ve got to get the darn cat out of him.”

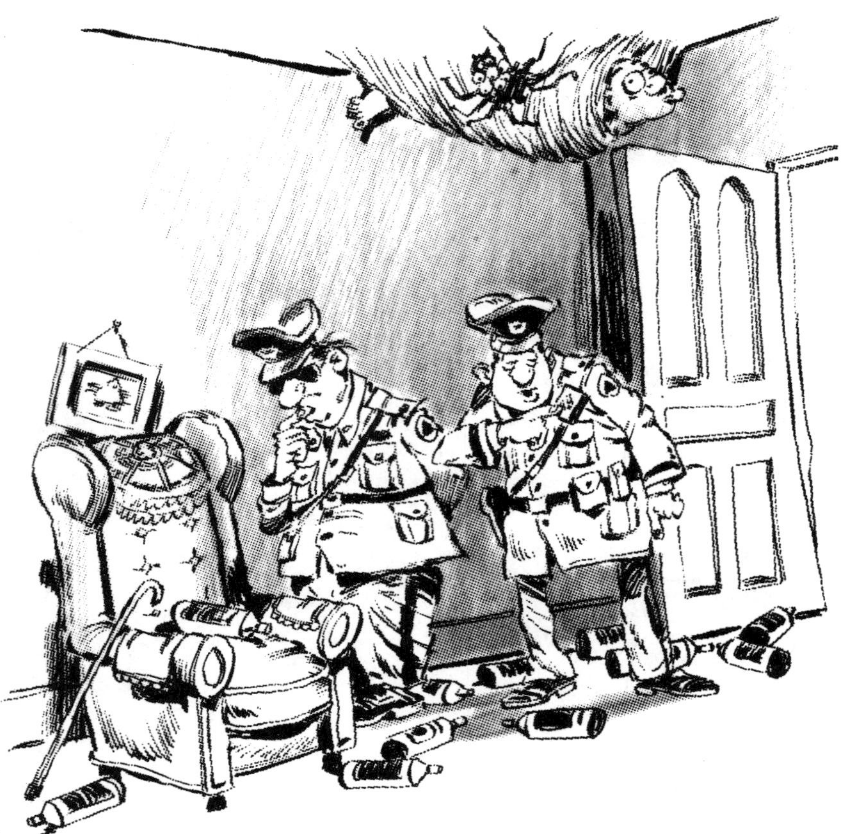

“....another prank call..nuttin’ here but a bunck of empty bug spray cans”

Here's lookin at cha............

We knew that this book would bring back a few memories of those that have shaped you into the A-1, First Class, Top Notch, Best of the Best, Worshiped and emulated Emergency Services Provider you are.......

Putting together these many attributes we have developed our conception of how these mentors would look if they were but one person.

You may be this person, want to be them or perhaps already know them,

The following pages will provide you with an inspirational graphic depiction of:

EMERGENCY SERVICES
HEROES and HEROINES

Official Autograph Page

Dear Super Medic,

As an influencing factor in my life. I would like you to sign my book.

This will assure that I will always have an official record that I know or knew you, and proof that you are in part responsible for making me what I am.

My lawyer has suggested that I obtain this signature for future reference should I be named in a legal proceeding.

Thank you,

________________________(you print your name here)

Please sign in ink.

____

____

____

____

____

____

____

____

____

THE PARAMEDIC

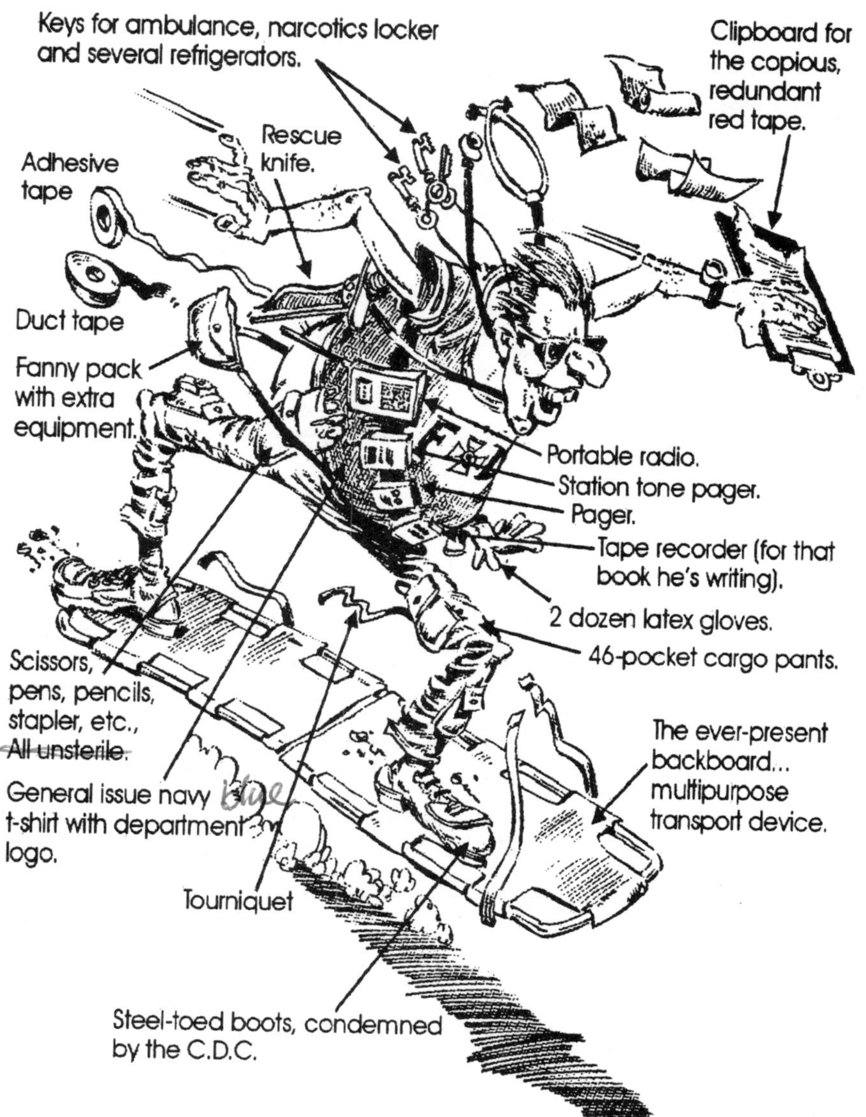

Official Autograph Page

Dear Super Nurse,

As an influencing factor in my life. I would like you to sign my book.

This will assure that I will always have an official record that I know or knew you, and proof that you are in part responsible for making me what I am.

My lawyer has suggested that I obtain this signature for future reference should I be named in a legal proceeding.

Thank you,

________________________(you print your name here)

Please sign in ink.

THE ER NURSE

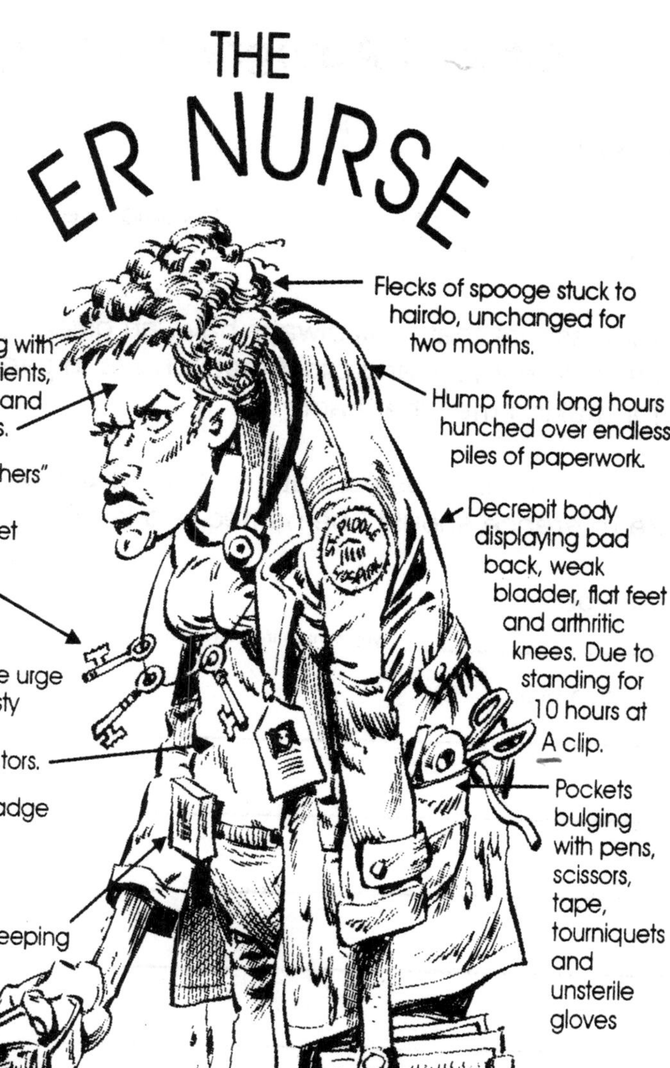

Permanent scowl from dealing with doctors, patients, ward clerks, and payroll clerks.
Flecks of spooge stuck to hairdo, unchanged for two months.
Hump from long hours hunched over endless piles of paperwork.
Keys to "leathers" (restraints), meds cabinet and ladies bathroom.
Decrepit body displaying bad back, weak bladder, flat feet and arthritic knees. Due to standing for 10 hours at A clip.
Ulcer from restraining the urge to punch nasty patients an d nastier doctors.
Pockets bulging with pens, scissors, tape, tourniquets and unsterile gloves
Hospital ID badge and listing of wearer's medications.
Continually beeping pager
Cheap, stained and smelly tennis shoes
Arms stretched to abnormal length from lifting patients, carrying charts and holding onto sanity.

Official Autograph Page

Dear Super Doc,

As an influencing factor in my life. I would like you to sign my book.

This will assure that I will always have an official record that I know or knew you, and proof that you are in part responsible for making me what I am.

My lawyer has suggested that I obtain this signature for future reference should I be named in a legal proceeding.

Thank you,

_________________________(you print your name here)

Please sign in ink.

____

____

____

____

____

____

____

____

____

THE ER INTERN

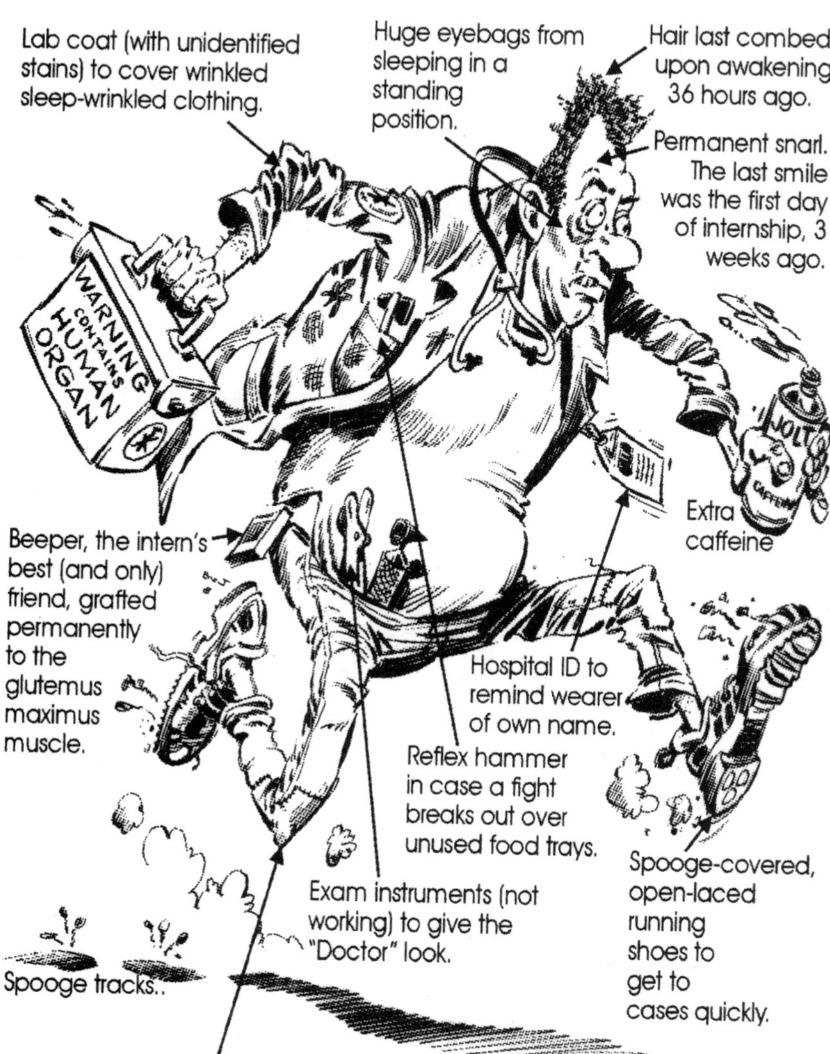

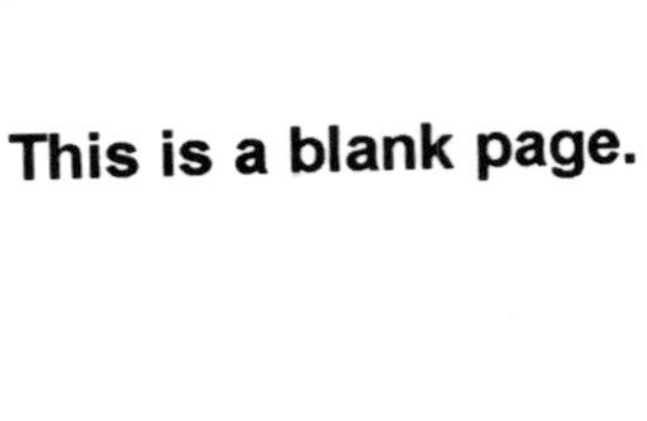

If you have purchased this book you can do what you want with this page.

If this book belongs to someone else you should return it immediately and buy your own copy.

Help Wanted
Emergency Services Workers

Firefighters, Rescue Squad Members, ER Nurses, Medics, Doctors and PoliceOfficers.

Must be able to work long hours for little or no pay. May be required to work frequent last minute mandatory overtime.

Few holidays and weekends off. Must be able to keep massive amounts of paperwork up to date while making split-second, life or death decisions.

Must be immune to verbal abuse and able to neutralize the occasional physical assault, up to and including armed a/o drugged attackers.

Ability to withstand lack of understanding and support from leadership, public and an abundance of internal and external arbitrary political "BS" is desiriable.

Must display patience, kindness, understanding and caring, even when personal life is coming apart at the seams. Must show no aversion to blood, vomit, oozing infections, or human body wastes.

This great oportunity to be understood and accepted by only your peers is yours for the asking.

Call Now, operators are standing by:

Local Fire Dept/ Rescue Squad	**Phone#**__________
Local Ambulance-EMS Service	**Phone#**__________
Local Hospital ER	**Phone#**__________
Local Police Department	**Phone#**__________

Instructions for use:
The above generic job announcement poster is provided for your convenience.

1.Cut off these instructions and write in the appropriate phone #(s)

2.Duplicate and post this announcement anywhere idealistic, naive individuals may see it.

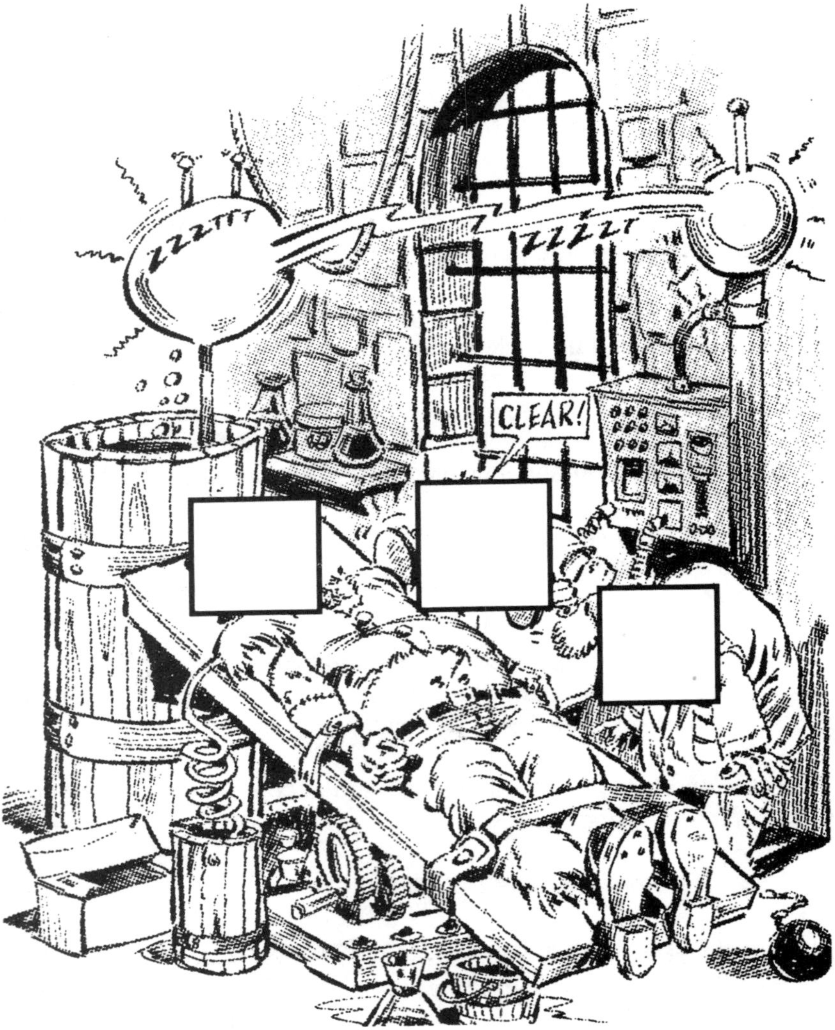

Self Study Promotional Exam

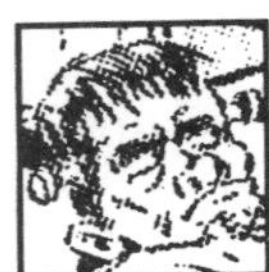

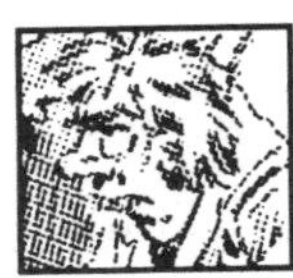

Paste your picture here

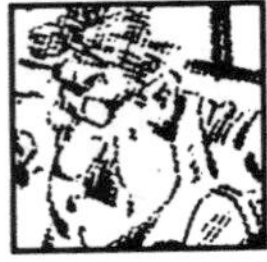

1. Paste your picture above.
2. Cut out all 4 small pictures
3. Place pictures in proper location's on above drawing.
4. Send copy to supervisor.